GARIBALDI SECONDARY SCHOOL
24789 Dewdney Trunk Road
Maple Ridge, B.C. V4R 1X2

DEADLY DISEASES AND EPIDEMICS

TOXIC SHOCK SYNDROME

Anthrax

Cholera

HIV/AIDS

Influenza

Lyme Disease

Malaria

Mononucleosis

Polio

Syphilis

Toxic Shock Syndrome

Tuberculosis

Typhoid Fever

DEADLY DISEASES AND EPIDEMICS

TOXIC SHOCK SYNDROME

Brian Shmaefsky

CONSULTING EDITOR
I. Edward Alcamo
Distinguished Teaching Professor of Microbiology,
SUNY Farmingdale

FOREWORD BY
David Heymann
World Health Organization

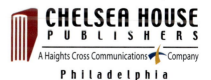

CHELSEA HOUSE
P U B L I S H E R S
A Haights Cross Communications Company
Philadelphia

Dedication

We dedicate the books in the DEADLY DISEASES AND EPIDEMICS series to Ed Alcamo, whose wit, charm, intelligence, and commitment to biology education were second to none.

CHELSEA HOUSE PUBLISHERS

VP, NEW PRODUCT DEVELOPMENT Sally Cheney
DIRECTOR OF PRODUCTION Kim Shinners
CREATIVE MANAGER Takeshi Takahashi
MANUFACTURING MANAGER Diann Grasse

Staff for Toxic Shock Syndrome

ASSOCIATE EDITOR Beth Reger
PRODUCTION EDITOR Megan Emery
PHOTO EDITOR Sarah Bloom
SERIES DESIGNER Terry Mallon
COVER DESIGNER Keith Trego
LAYOUT 21st Century Publishing and Communications, Inc.

http://www.chelseahouse.com

First Printing

1 3 5 7 9 8 6 4 2

Library of Congress Cataloging-in-Publication Data

Shmaefsky, Brian.
  Toxic shock syndrome/by Brian R. Shmaefsky.
    p. cm.—(Your body, how it works)
Includes bibliographical references and index.
Contents: A new disease—Toxic shock syndrome—Septic diseases: the body defends itself—Staphylococcus and stss—Streptococcus and streptss—Epidemiology—Diagnosis and treatment.
  ISBN 0-7910-7465-X
  1. Toxic shock syndrome—Juvenile literature. [1. Toxic shock syndrome.]
I. Title. II. Series.
RG220.S564 2003
616.9'297—dc22

                                                                2003016778

Table of Contents

Foreword

In the 1960s, infectious diseases—which had terrorized generations—
were tamed. Building on a century of discoveries, the leading killers
of Americans both young and old were being prevented with new
vaccines or cured with new medicines. The risk of death from
pneumonia, tuberculosis, meningitis, influenza, whooping cough,
and diphtheria declined dramatically. New vaccines lifted the fear
that summer would bring polio, and a global campaign was
approaching the global eradication of smallpox. New pesticides
like DDT cleared mosquitoes from homes and fields, thus reducing
the incidence of malaria which was present in the southern United
States and a leading killer of children worldwide. New technologies
produced safe drinking water and removed the risk of cholera and
other water-borne diseases. Science seemed unstoppable. Disease
seemed destined to almost disappear.

But the euphoria of the 1960s has evaporated.

Microbes fight back. Those causing diseases like TB and malaria
evolved resistance to cheap and effective drugs. The mosquito evolved
the ability to defuse pesticides. New diseases emerged, including
AIDS, Legionnaires, and Lyme disease. And diseases which have not
been seen in decades re-emerge, as the hantavirus did in the Navajo
Nation in 1993. Technology itself actually created new health risks.
The global transportation network, for example, meant that diseases
like West Nile virus could spread beyond isolated regions in distant
countries and quickly become global threats. Even modern public
health protections sometimes failed, as they did in Milwaukee,
Wisconsin in 1993 which resulted in 400,000 cases of the digestive
system illness cryptosporidiosis. And, more recently, the threat from
smallpox, a disease completely eradicated, has returned along with
other potential bioterrorism weapons such as anthrax.

The lesson is that the fight against infectious diseases will
never end.

In this constant struggle against disease, we as individuals have
a weapon that does not require vaccines or drugs, the warehouse
of knowledge. We learn from the history of science that "modern"
beliefs can be wrong. In this series of books, for example, you will

learn that diseases like syphilis were once thought to be caused by eating potatoes. The invention of the microscope set science on the right path. There are more positive lessons from history. For example, smallpox was eliminated by vaccinating everyone who had come in contact with an infected person. This "ring" approach to controlling smallpox is still the preferred method for confronting a smallpox outbreak should the disease be intentionally reintroduced.

At the same time, we are constantly adding new drugs, new vaccines, and new information to the warehouse. Recently, the entire human genome was decoded. So too was the genome of the parasite that causes malaria. Perhaps by looking at the microbe and the victim through the lens of genetics we will to be able to discover new ways of fighting malaria, still the leading killer of children in many countries.

Because of the knowledge gained about such diseases as AIDS, entire new classes of anti-retroviral drugs have been developed. But resistance to all these drugs has already been detected, so we know that AIDS drug development must continue.

Education, experimentation, and the discoveries which grow out of them are the best tools to protect health. Opening this book may put you on the path of discovery. I hope so, because new vaccines, new antibiotics, new technologies and, most importantly, new scientists are needed now more than ever if we are to remain on the winning side of this struggle with microbes.

David Heymann
Executive Director
Communicable Diseases Section
World Health Organization
Geneva, Switzerland

1

A "New" Disease

Nothing happens quite by chance. It's a question of accretion of information and experience.

Jonas Salk, microbiologist, 1914–1995

Chance works together with knowledge of the past when unearthing the unexplained **outbreak** of a **disease. Toxic shock syndrome** was an obscure disease limited to a particular population of people in which the disease predictably appeared. Thus, people did little to explore the disease fully. In addition, they may have erroneously interpreted the spread of many cases because they thought that the disease had only one way of entering the body. It took an outbreak in an unexpected population of people to make the medical community rethink the way toxic shock syndrome could occur. The severity of the new outbreak and the public fear fueled by intensive media coverage hastened efforts to understand this new disorder.

Symptoms of toxic shock syndrome have been documented as early as the ancient Greeks. Hippocrates (Figure 1.1), the Greek physician who lived about 460–377 B.C., was the first to record a condition called erysipelas, which medical historians believe might have been toxic shock syndrome. Hippocrates' studies on injured people documented cases in which " . . . the erysipelas would quickly spread in all directions." In his accounts, he added that large patches of skin, muscle, and tendon fell away from the bones. In the 1900s, it quickly became a disease associated with **trauma** from automobile accidents, industrial mishaps, and war injuries.

Hippocrates' description of erysipelas was similar to the indications of the most recent toxic shock outbreak in the early 1980s, which gained public recognition of the disease. However, the severity of

8

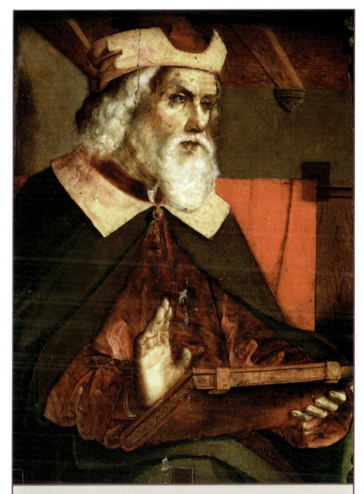

Figure 1.1 The Greek physician Hippocrates, shown here, was the first to record an outbreak of erysipelas, or what may have been toxic shock syndrome. Toxic shock syndrome remained a relatively rare disease until an outbreak in the 1980s, which was linked to the use of a certain brand of tampons.

the disease back in his time had a lot to do with a lack of medical treatment. In addition, a weakened immune response due to the primeval lifestyles aggravated the disease. For the disease to become common and severe in modern times was unexpected. After all, one would assume that healthier living environments and better access to medicine would lessen the impact of disease. However, a new category of conditions called **emergent diseases** seems to be taking advantage of contemporary living conditions. They take advantage of unknown or incompletely understood opportunities to cause disease. Many factors related to the development of human civilization lead to the onset of emergent diseases. Toxic shock syndrome was classified as an emergent disease when it was found to be associated with certain feminine hygiene practices.

CASE HISTORY OF AN EMERGENT DISEASE
Toxic shock syndrome came to the forefront of medical discussion with its emergence in association with female menstrual hygiene practices. This emergence is illustrated with

NEW EMERGENT DISEASES

Emergent diseases such as toxic shock syndrome are mentioned all the time in the news. SARS, sudden acute respiratory syndrome, and monkey pox made their way into international headlines in 2003. SARS spread rapidly through Asia, making its way to North America and Europe leaving dozens of dead people in every community it struck. The severe respiratory disease is caused by a new form of the common cold virus. Scientists believe it arose from contact with animals that carried this changed form of the cold virus. The animals developed the disease because of the crowded conditions used to store the live animals before slaughter. The close contact between animals and people selling the animals caused many humans to develop the disease. Monkey pox was brought to the United States by the sale of African rats with the virus. The virus quickly infected other rodent pets and started spreading a mild disease to humans. Luckily, the monkey pox virus is not fatal in humans.

the following case study, presented by Dr. Regina LaRocque, speaking at an **infectious**-disease conference in 2001.

> L.F. is a 37-year-old woman without significant past medical history who presented to an outside hospital with fever, rash, and malaise. Two days prior to admission, the patient awoke with nausea followed by profuse bilious vomiting and loose stools. Concomitantly, she noted a new rash in the folds of her groin. The rash subsequently progressed to involve her trunk and extremities and was later associated with sore throat and fever.

So far, the description above given in the notes handed out to the audience could have been explaining a host of bacterial and viral diseases that commonly afflict humans. The story further unfolded to reveal more about this severe disease.

> The patient presented to an outside emergency department, where she was found to have a temperature of 104.5, blood pressure of 80/58, and tachycardia [increased heart rate] to the 130s. On exam, she was ill-appearing but alert and oriented. Her skin exam was remarkable for a diffuse blanching erythematous [red] rash most prominent in the groin and lower abdomen. HEENT exam [a type of physical exam] revealed conjunctival injection as well as erythema [reddening] of the posterior oropharynx [back of the mouth]. Her neck was supple, and there was no lymphadenopathy [swelling of the tonsils].

This continued elaboration of the condition, as confusing as it is to the common person, put a distinct fear in those who had the knowledge to figure out the condition. The audience listened intently as LaRocque recounted what they now knew was the uncommon toxic shock syndrome.

LaRocque's presentation brought back memories of a report published in 1980 by the Centers for Disease Control and Prevention (CDC) in Atlanta, Georgia. The CDC advised medical professionals and public health officials to look for an outbreak of toxic shock syndrome. The report stated:

> Cases of newly recognized illness known as toxic-shock syndrome have recently been reported to CDC by state health departments in Wisconsin, Minnesota, Illinois, Utah, and Idaho. Physicians in 8 other states have reported individual cases to CDC or to investigators at the University of Colorado, Denver.

It went on to describe how doctors reported 55 cases in 1979 with 95 percent of the cases occurring in women. The report also explained that the disease was more likely in women 13–52 years old. It killed 13 percent of the people who sought medical care. LaRocque's description of L.F. echoed the cases mentioned in the report that came out 22 years before L.F.'s affliction. The doctor diagnosed L.F. with the condition toxic shock syndrome, classified in 1979 as an emergent disease. Emergent diseases such as toxic shock syndrome have steadily plagued people with growth and progress of human civilization (Figure 1.2).

HISTORY OF EMERGENT DISEASES

Ancient civilizations and nomadic peoples usually made few records of devastating diseases. This outward gap in history was not due to a lapse in recording disease and suffering. The opposite was true. Historical records have many accounts of disease described in precise detail. Disease was very important in early times, oddly, because of the social stigmas equated with disease. In many cultures, disease was equated with inherited weaknesses, lewdness, filthiness, gluttony, sin, and slovenliness. However, some cultures kept good records for the moral education of their people. The number of diseases reported in history appeared to rise with the development of civilization and a subsequent increase in agricultural practices, exploration, population growth, recreation, technology, and **urbanization.**

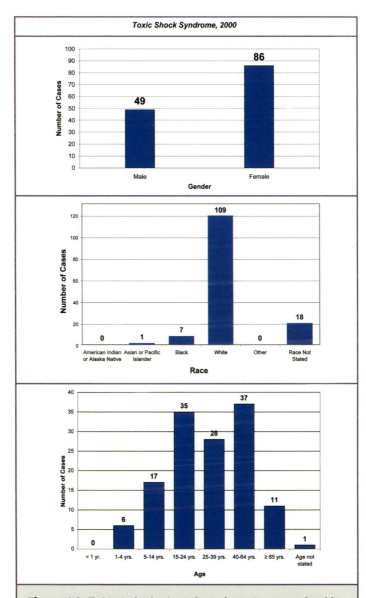

Figure 1.2 Today, toxic shock syndrome is most common in white women between the ages of 15 and 65, as can be seen on the three graphs here. Toxic shock syndrome occurs more frequently in women as it has been linked to tampon use. Among the surveyed groups, American Indians and native Alaskans had the fewest incidences of the disease.

Agriculture was a natural outcome of human civilization. Civilization brought with it the permanent settlement of areas rich in resources. Years of living in a region compounded by an increasing population led to a reduction of animals and plants for food. Consequently, this forced people to rely less on traditional foraging and hunting practices. They had to **domesticate** and raise the animals and plants needed for sustenance. This produced a situation in which people were living in close contact with the domesticated animals. Immediately after the domestication of animals came the onset of previously unknown human ailments. Only recently have we discovered that these diseases came from the domesticated animals. For example, we now know that the common childhood disease **pink eye** (conjunctivitis) originated in cattle. It still causes a related eye **infection** in dairy and milk cows. The notorious disease **smallpox**, in addition to a host of other widespread human ailments, was at one time limited to animals. Even today, domesticated animals are the source of new human diseases. An article published in the January 2003 issue of the scientific journal *Trends in Parasitology* reported how an infectious **protozoan** called *Leishmania* passed from wild animals to dogs and then to humans. Another study in the same journal is investigating the probable spread of a cattle protozoan disease to dogs and possibly humans.

Along with civilization came the exploration of new land to offset the crowding caused by rapid population growth in ancient towns and metropolitan areas. Food shortages became commonplace as agriculture and natural resources could not keep up with the growing population's needs. People migrated to new areas to exploit the untapped resources. New areas brought exposure to new **microorganisms** that inhabited the local animals and soils. For example, the colonization of Europe from Africa introduced people to flu (influenza), measles, and tuberculosis. The highly destructive Ebola **virus** and the human immunodeficiency virus (HIV), which causes acquired immune deficiency syndrome (AIDS), may relate

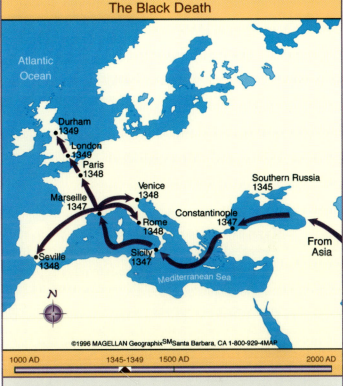

Figure 1.3 Many diseases emerge as people travel to and from different areas of the world. The black plague (also known as the Black Death), for example, was introduced to Europe by traders and travelers returning from Asia (as can be seen on the map shown here). Europeans had never experienced this disease before, and thus were very susceptible and unable to fend off the illness.

to human settlement of remote forests in Africa. Various **encephalitis** viruses, some of which are currently plaguing the United States, are believed to come from living in close contact with birds of the forest. Exploration also became a way of introducing emergent diseases into new areas. For example, human migration introduced **black plague** to Europe through trade with Asia (Figure 1.3). Europeans brought their emergent diseases to the Americas, killing many of the indigenous peoples.

Areas of the Middle East and North America in ancient times had the same overpopulation problems of modern cities. Crime, overcrowded housing, pollution, and poverty abounded. With these problems came the appearance of new diseases. Overcrowding in cities creates two factors that encourage the development of emergent diseases. First, it allows the buildup of wastes and litter that attract insects and rodents. This puts people in regular contact with microorganisms living on the pests. These microorganisms can then spread to people, causing previously unknown diseases. Second, overcrowding makes it easier for diseases to spread from one person to another. This allowed new diseases to gain a foothold in the human population by being able to jump readily to uninfected people. In rural areas, the diseases could not spread and simply died out with the infected people. Exploration and migrations to other populated areas further spread diseases.

The following excerpt from the CRC's *Handbook of Marine Mammal Medicine,* published in 2001, reveals one avenue for creating new human diseases.

> Reports of the transmission of disease from marine mammals to humans are scarce; however, as humans are increasingly in contact with marine mammals, the possibility of encountering new disease must be considered. Lack of reports in the literature may indicate lack of occurrence of disease, but may also reflect lack of recognition by physicians or failure to report for a variety of reasons. Until recently, only hunters and scientists were likely to have close physical contact with marine mammals, and the public's exposure was limited to zoos or aquaria with animals behind barriers. However, in the last decade, human contact with marine mammals has changed so that a broader range of people are exposed to zoonoses.

Increased exposure to marine mammals is related to the increasing popularity of boating, scuba diving, surfing, and swimming. Improvement in zoos makes for better contact with humans and animals, because the animals are less confined and are closer to people. Ecotourism can also be to blame, because more and more people are taking vacations that bring them in contact with marine mammals. Thus, the stage is set for the better transmission of disease between people and marine mammals (**zoonoses**), making real the possibility of new emergent diseases. Early in human history, hunting may have predisposed people to emergent diseases, as it does today with conditions such as **Lyme disease.**

EFFECTS OF TECHNOLOGY

In some opinions, technology was intended to free people from the capricious forces and limitations of nature. Machines were designed to alleviate wear and tear on the body from heavy manual labor. Processed food would make it safer and simpler for people to feed a family. Comfortable housing was developed to protect people from ailments due to exposure to the weather. Most important to relieving human suffering was the advent of modern medical practices, including refined medications and precise **therapeutic** techniques. Medicine and hygiene would ease suffering and prevent disease. Early in human history, it did so and helped people to reach unprecedented population growth by decreasing the chance of dying young.

Unfortunately, what helped humans also provided a means for emergent diseases to develop. The machines that made life easier have predisposed people to new infectious disease. Sedentary lifestyles have resulted from technologies that reduced manual labor. With this inactivity has come a general decline in health such as obesity and weaker cardiovascular systems. The technology also has produced loads of industrial wastes that pollute the air and the water. Combined with diets high in processed foods, these factors make the body more susceptible to infectious diseases. **Microbes** that normally live on the body without causing harm can produce disease if the body becomes weak from a lack of fitness and health. Housing created tightly enclosed environments that trapped and concentrated infectious microbes. People started receiving higher dosages of microbes from each other, pets, and household pests such as cockroaches, mice, and rats. This set up the conditions for increase in diseases that were normally unheard-of and rare.

How medicine and hygiene created more susceptibility to emergent diseases surprised the medical community. **Antibiotics** cured people of bacterial diseases, yet they also led to exposure to new infections. As antibiotics killed one disease, another appeared to replace it. Scientists discovered that unknown **pathogens** were not getting a chance to cause disease as more common ailments obscured them. In addition, the continued use of antibiotics led to **antibiotic-resistant** bacteria. Bacteria carrying **traits** making them unaffected by antibiotics replaced those killed by the medications. Thus came a host of emergent diseases known as antibiotic-resistant infections. Improved personal hygiene created other problems. It limited human exposure to many microbes, rendering the **immune system** uninitiated to persistent infection. Thus, people now become ill more easily from common microbes that do not readily cause disease. Although hygienic practices such as sewage treatment removed hazardous bacteria, sanitary items such as diapers and feminine-hygiene products kept microbes in contact with the body. This continued contact created new diseases caused by skin bacteria, including toxic shock syndrome.

Surgery and medical devices were as equally responsible as antibiotics for introducing emergent diseases into the human population. Bacteria that enters the body through surgery and through the insertion of tubes into body openings creates new types of diseases. Many people who receive **urinary-tract catheters** develop infections that are sometimes aggressive and very difficult to treat. Even simple tasks, such as cosmetic surgery, have created problems with unexpected bacterial infections. Several people who have received artificial implants or have undergone liposuction have contracted unusual diseases that could have readily spread throughout hospitals if vigilant medical intervention had not caught and contained them.

Lastly, urbanization alone paved the way for new diseases to emerge in the human population. The development of urban areas created crowded living conditions unknown to ancient people. With crowding comes the increased transmission of disease between people and from animals to people. Crowded living conditions in Medieval Europe aided in the spread of black plague. By living in close contact with rats, people were very susceptible to rat fleabites. People then had more exposure to the plague bacterium, *Yersinia pestis*, permitting it to establish disease in humans, as the bacterium is carried by fleas from rats to humans. Crowding thus encouraged the spread of black plague directly throughout the human population. History shows that ancient urban centers in Egypt were home to some of the earliest known emergent diseases. Still haunting humans is smallpox, which presented itself in 1600 B.C.; mumps, dating to 400 B.C.; and **leprosy**, which became prevalent in 200 B.C. Urbanization in nineteenth-century Europe was considered responsible for the establishment of **polio**.

Henceforth, toxic shock syndrome belongs to a large group of diseases represented by ancient and modern conditions that accompanied humans with the development of civilization. Toxic shock syndrome most likely started out as an exotic disease associated with war injuries or other extreme traumas. This basis of toxic shock syndrome dates to 400 B.C. Surgery and other **invasive treatments** became the next cause of toxic shock syndrome, as researchers reported cases with the advent of each new medical procedure. Then, in the 1970s, it became evident that new feminine hygiene practices introduced a different means for producing toxic shock syndrome. Luckily, a keen watchfulness for emergent diseases led the medical community to the rapid identification of this novel way of contracting the disease.

2

Toxic Shock Syndrome

The pain of the mind is worse than the pain of the body.

Publius Syrus, circa 100 A.D.

Few who suffered from toxic shock syndrome would agree with Syrus. The bodily pain surely is more miserable than the agony of a lost love or an athletic defeat. Body aches, **fever**, a painful rash, and a host of other problems accompany toxic shock syndrome. Ironically, it is the relative of a safe bacterium that causes the more common form of this insidious ailment. **Bacteria** are microscopic **organisms** composed of a single, simple **cell**. Most bacteria do not affect humans. However, some are beneficial whereas others cause disease. Relatives of the bacterium that causes toxic shock syndrome normally colonize the skin and **respiratory system**, protecting the body from infections.

The suffering of people with toxic shock syndrome went virtually unnoticed until the disease gained widespread public attention in the 1980s. The profusion of news broadcasts announcing the apparent "new plague" caught the public off-guard. It was a complex disease caused by mundane activities related to feminine hygiene practices. In addition, a little-known bacterium called **Staphylococcus aureus**, recognized mostly for causing skin irritations, caused the common form of the disease (Figure 2.1). Women in particular were frightened because they fit into the highest risk category of getting toxic shock syndrome because of the disease's link to feminine hygiene.

Luckily, swift action by various physicians and by the CDC allayed public fear by identifying the disease and bringing it under control. Most important was promptly finding preventive measures based on

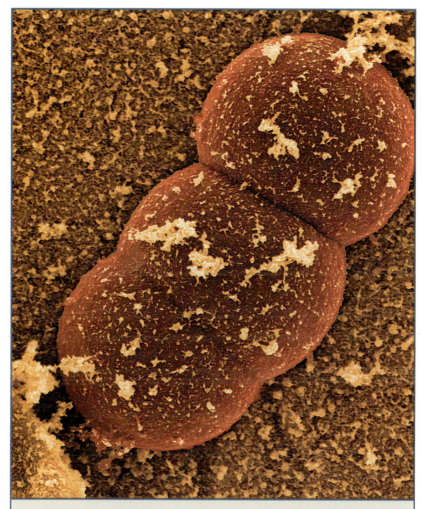

Figure 2.1 *Staphylococcus aureus* is a type of bacteria that causes toxic shock syndrome. The bacteria are spherical in shape, and usually clump together. An electron micrograph of *Staphylococcus aureus* is shown here.

understanding the cause of the disease. At first, researchers connected only *Staphylococcus aureus* with toxic shock syndrome. *Staphylococcus aureus* was a pathogen known throughout the medical literature to cause similar maladies.

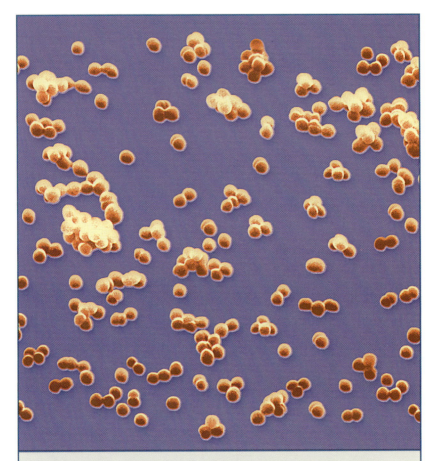

Figure 2.2 *Streptococcus pyogenes* also causes toxic shock syndrome. An electron micrograph of the bacteria is shown here. Like *Staphylococcus aureus*, *Streptococcus pyogenes* are spherical bacteria and usually clump together in a chain (although some larger clusters are also apparent).

Another form of toxic shock syndrome appeared later. The disease, almost indistinguishable from toxic shock, was caused by **Streptococcus pyogenes**, another known pathogenic bacterium (Figure 2.2). Both of these bacteria have wide genetic variety, making it difficult to predict the severity of disease that they can cause.

The diseases that they cause, collectively called toxic shock, have a common thread. It entails bodily decay due to invading bacteria that produce toxic **secretions**. The secretions do their evil deeds solely for the survival of the bacteria. Some secretions permit the bacteria to feed upon its **host**'s body whereas others protect the bacteria from the body's defenses. Unfortunately, the consequence of the invasion leads to a set of **signs** and **symptoms** that can lead to permanent body damage or death, known as toxic shock syndrome.

THE DISEASE

Toxic shock syndrome fittingly earns the name "**syndrome**" in its title. This term refers to diseases that cause a variety of ailments. Syndromes are not limited to one identifiable problem leading physicians to a simple **diagnosis**. Toxic shock syndrome is composed of a variety of signs and symptoms that collectively point a medical doctor to the condition. The term *sign* refers to conditions that physicians can measure and see. Examples of signs include fever or rash. Each sign alone tells a story about the specific effects of the disease on the body. For example, a rash can indicate an **allergy** to the organism or a response to irritating secretions produced by the organism. *Symptoms* are subjective indications of a disease. Physicians cannot measure symptoms. Nonetheless, symptoms can indicate whether disease is present. Examples of symptoms include conditions reported by the patient, such as headache and body pains.

Unfortunately for the medical community, toxic shock syndrome presents a variety of signs and symptoms resembling other diseases. The condition is in fact just an indication that bacteria have breached the body's defenses and have invaded the bloodstream and other organs. Many patients show most of the signs and symptoms associated with toxic shock syndrome, but others exhibit only a few. Its signs consist of bleeding, bruising, diarrhea, difficulty breathing, fever, low blood pressure, rash, reddening of the mouth and urinary tract, shedding of the skin, skin infections, and vomiting. Physicians normally find a loss of liver function as the disease progresses. Symptoms of toxic shock syndrome include chills, discomfort, disorientation, fatigue, headache, muscle pains, and nausea. The disease generally causes hospitalization and death if untreated.

Staphylococcal toxic shock syndrome has signs and symptoms similar to those of **streptococcal toxic shock syndrome**. However, they mostly differ in the degree to which each ailment appears. What both have in common is that all patients show fever, a drop in blood pressure, and the chance of going into **shock**. Research studies show that 90–100 percent of people with staphylococcal toxic shock also have diarrhea, disorientation, reddening of the skin, and vomiting. In some patients, the fever may exceed 104°F or 40°C. Headaches and muscle aches are also common in most cases of staphylococcal toxic shock syndrome. Breathing difficulties are a general indication of the infection.

Only 20–25 percent of people with streptococcal toxic shock syndrome develop discomfort, disorientation, and nausea. Less than 10 percent complain of headaches. However, over half of the afflicted people say that they have muscle pains. Vomiting occurs in about 25 percent of the cases, and breathing difficulties arise in less than 10 percent of the people infected with toxic shock bacteria. Reddening of the skin is not always present.

Initially, physicians may misinterpret toxic shock syndrome as flu, which is caused by an unrelated organism called the influenza virus. Doctors exclude flu as a diagnosis as the disease progresses beyond the normal range of ailments associated with an influenza infection. Then it can be confused with a wide variety of diseases, including **leptospirosis**, measles, and **Rocky Mountain spotted fever**. Leptospirosis is an intestinal disease caused by the **spirochete** bacterium *Leptospira*, obtained from cooking and drinking water contaminated with animal and human urine. An infectious virus called rubeola causes measles. Rocky Mountain spotted fever is caused by a bacterium spread by the bites of certain lice, mites, and ticks. Doctors exclude these other diseases after they run laboratory tests that identify the offending organism.

Toxic shock syndrome gets its start when *Staphylococcus aureus* or *Streptococcus pyogenes* gains entrance to the body. In many cases, it occurs when unusually large amounts of bacteria overgrow and irritate **mucous membranes**. Under normal conditions, mucous membranes protect the body from pathogens, or disease-causing organisms. However, when aggravated by disease, the mucous membranes will allow pathogens to enter the body. Bacteria can also enter the body through open wounds. The pathogens causing toxic shock syndrome produce secretions that help the bacteria enter the body. In many cases, all they need is a chance to get on the surface of the body in enough numbers for a few to pass by the body's defenses successfully. This entry stage usually does not create any problems for the victim. Signs and symptoms of the disease usually do not appear until the bacteria have gotten a foothold in the body.

It usually takes about 3 to 7 days after bacterial invasion for the signs and symptoms of toxic shock syndrome to appear. Public awareness about the diseases occurred from an unexpected route of invasion and infection. Many cases of toxic shock syndrome in the 1980s appeared to start in the vaginal tract (Figure 2.3), due to *Staphylococcus aureus* growing on improperly used **tampons**. Other incidents of staphylococcal toxic shock syndrome resulted from burns, respiratory diseases, and skin wounds, all which allowed the bacteria to easily enter the body. Streptococcal toxic shock syndrome may accompany or follow AIDS, chickenpox, and serious skin infections. Skin wounds resulting from accidents and battle injuries can readily lead to either *Staphylococcus aureus* or *Streptococcus pyogenes* invasion.

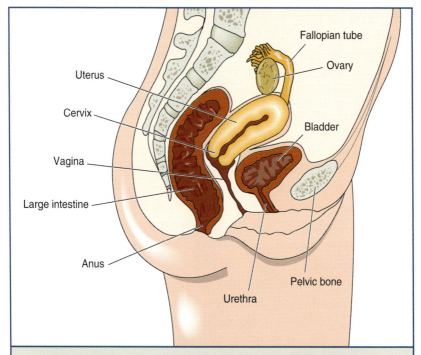

Figure 2.3 The common form of toxic shock syndrome seen in the 1980s began as vaginal tract infections. Many cases were linked to the use of a certain brand of tampons. The bacteria that cause TSS like warm, moist environments such as the vaginal tract, illustrated here, which provides an optimal location for bacterial replication.

The first indication of both forms of toxic shock syndrome (caused by either *Staphylococcus aureus* or *Streptococcus pyogenes*) is redness and irritation at the point of entry. However, this is not evident in most cases of the disease, and many times the symptoms are minimal or go unnoticed. At this point in the disease, bacterial secretions are inflaming the skin and may even be making it easier for the bacteria to gain their way through skin and mucous membrane barriers. Next, body temperature rises to about 102°F or 38.9°C. Both diseases show a rapid onset of fever followed by occurrence of the other signs and symptoms. The fever also results from bacterial secretions.

At this point in the disease, the bacterial secretions are in the blood, causing the whole body to respond to the invasion. The symptoms also start at this point. Chills, discomfort, and fatigue result from the fever. Further differences in the symptoms result from the type of bacterium invading the body and from individual differences among people. Other body responses to infection are due to the different bacteria causing the disease and the place where the bacteria entered the body.

THE ORGANISM
Staphylococcus aureus

As previously mentioned in this chapter, *Staphylococcus aureus* was the first bacterium noted for causing toxic shock syndrome. It is incorrect to state that it produces the most potent form of toxic shock syndrome, given that it kills only 3 percent of those with the disease. However, the disease is abrupt and does lead to the most severe signs and symptoms. It is obvious when people have the *Staphylococcus* form of toxic shock syndrome because of the high incidence of ailments associated with the bacterial invasion. *Staphylococcus aureus* belongs to group of bacteria normally found on the skin, throughout the respiratory system, in the large intestine, and in parts of the female **reproductive tract**. The organism causes little harm unless it overgrows or passes through the skin into the body.

The organism is a spherical bacterium that grows in highly branching clumps. *Staphylococcus aureus* is no stranger to the body. According to medical studies, more than 90 percent of the people in North America have had exposure to *Staphylococcus aureus*. Few people with *Staphylococcus aureus* actively growing on the body show any indication of disease. Most scientists believe that *Staphylococcus aureus* is more likely to cause disease in people susceptible to an invasive infection. This includes people suffering from infected skin wounds and those with immune systems weakened by ailing health.

Not all **strains** of *Staphylococcus aureus* cause disease in humans. The ability to produce disease depends mainly on genetic differences between several varieties or strains of *Staphylococcus aureus*. In addition, the presence of the bacterium is not the actual cause of disease. A particular group of bacterial secretions called **exotoxins** assist with bacterial survival in the host. One group of exotoxins, called **superantigens**, creates the disease condition in staphylococcal toxic shock syndrome. **Enterotoxins** are another type of superantigen. They generally reside in the digestive system of the pathogen's host. Bacteria that produce disease through a particular secretion that affects the host are termed **intoxicants. Infectants** are bacteria whose sole presence produces disease. The chemistry of their cell structure and survival activities creates disease.

A superantigen called **TSST-1**, or toxic shock syndrome toxin 1, produces disease in 75 percent of the staphylococcal toxic shock syndrome cases. Enterotoxin B occurs in another 23 percent of cases, whereas enterotoxin C causes approximately 2 percent of the staphylococcal toxic shock syndrome cases diagnosed. These superantigens affect the body by overstimulating the host's immune system. They interact with an immune system cell called the T cell. T cells produce a variety of their own secretions, all of which set in motion bodily events meant to fight off infection. However, superantigens produce a condition in which the body's immune system cells accidentally damage the body.

Again, it is the host's immune response to the superantigens that produce the signs of staphylococcal toxic shock syndrome. The chemistry of the superantigens does not directly harm the body like many other bacteria secretions. T cell secretions called interleukins stimulated by the superantigens produce the fever normally found with an infection. The extreme fever noted in staphylococcal toxic shock syndrome is due to the superantigen's ability to induce T cells to overproduce interleukins. Eventually, the superantigens produce a condition similar to **autoimmune disease**, in which the body accidentally uses the immune system to attack itself. This brings out the other signs and symptoms of staphylococcal toxic shock syndrome. Most typical of autoimmune responses to infection are the rashes and soreness. Also evident is the "scalded skin" appearance, resulting from the death of skin and subsequent rapid shedding of skin cells (Figure 2.4).

The shock component of staphylococcal toxic shock syndrome can occur when the weakened body fails to keep the person conscious. Low blood pressure and the loss of liver function are the major contributors to shock. Watery diarrhea can also be a factor in shock by reducing the amount of salts in the body needed to run muscles and the nervous system.

ALLERGIC RESPONSES

The allergic response that causes the skin rash in toxic shock syndrome is common with other types of diseases. Many people who suffer from allergies will develop rashes on the skin and internal organs when exposed to disease organisms. People with extreme allergies, or hypersensitivities, can get a rash by contact with certain animals and plants. This contact can be from handling a certain type of pet to eating a particular food. Many people with food allergies first suffer from abdominal pains before developing a mild skin rash called urticaria. Physicians have to conduct a variety of blood tests to determine the cause of urticaria. Allergists are physicians who specialize in finding and treating the causes of allergies. Not all people show an allergic response, even to the toxins produced during toxic shock syndrome. For some reason their immune systems do not react to the certain molecules contaminating the body. They might not suffer from the rash ailments, but they run the risk that septic diseases and other conditions could go unnoticed until they get deathly ill.

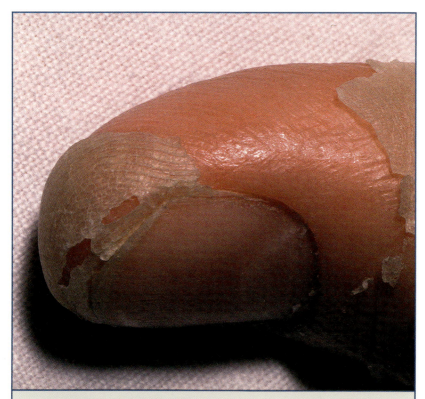

Figure 2.4 The reddened and shedding skin characteristic (also known as "scalded skin") of toxic shock syndrome is due to the body's overreaction to bacterial superantigens. The person whose thumb is shown in this picture is suffering from toxic shock syndrome. The disease kills skin cells, which the body rapidly sheds.

Streptococcus pyogenes

Streptococcus pyogenes, like *Staphylococcus aureus*, is an intoxicant pathogen that produces disease with its exotoxin secretions. However, the similarity stops here. *Streptococcus pyogenes* not only differs in appearance from *Staphylococcus aureus* but it also produces different types of exotoxins, which create a characteristic syndrome as the disease progresses. *Streptococcus pyogenes* grows as a straight chain of spherical bacterial cells. This organism became the explanation for many incidents of toxic shock syndrome not attributed to *Staphylococcus aureus* infections in animals and humans.

Bacteria related to *Streptococcus pyogenes* are common inhabitants of the body. Their presence assists with a variety of functions ranging from aiding in digestion to protecting against invasion by pathogenic bacteria and **fungi**. Many types of pathogenic streptococci cause disease in animals and humans, however. *Streptococcus pyogenes* is one of the more severe pathogenic forms. The difference between being beneficial and causing disease lies in the types of secretions produced by the different types of bacteria.

Streptococcus pyogenes produces a greater variety of toxins than *Staphylococcus aureus*. These compounds produce a wider array of damage to the host. *Streptococcus pyogenes* belongs to a group of streptococci called Group A Streptococci, or GAS. Streptolysin O and exotoxin B are two of its secretions that destroy host cells, setting up the body for damage and stimulating an immune response. Part of the immune response includes the release of body chemicals called tumor necrosis factors, which destroy host cells. This eventually leads to organ failure. Certain hormones also add to the pathogenic abilities of *Streptococcus pyogenes*. Other exotoxins, called **pyrogenic** toxins, produce the heightened fever noted in streptococcal toxic shock syndrome. **Enzymes** secreted by *Streptococcus pyogenes* also permit it to cause disease. These enzymes digest the host's **tissues**, permitting *Streptococcus pyogenes* to enter the body and feed upon the host's tissues.

A unique characteristic of *Streptococcus pyogenes* allows it to evade the body's defenses against bacterial invasion. A chemical called M protein covers *Streptococcus pyogenes*. M protein makes *Streptococcus pyogenes* a potent pathogen by protecting it from destruction by cells of the host's immune system. With this protein coating, it can spread through the body almost without interference. This bacterium is more persistent than *Staphylococcus aureus*. In turn, it does more damage to the body and can kill 30 percent of treated patients. The unrelenting spread of the bacteria causes most of the shock component of streptococcal toxic shock syndrome. Unlike staphylococcal toxic shock syndrome, shock and further illness relate less to the diarrhea and vomiting. In many cases, the bacteria start eating away the flesh and internal organs, leading to a condition called necrotizing disease.

CONCLUSION

Toxic shock syndrome is an incredible disease created by the body attacking itself in response to an infection. There are two identified forms of toxic shock, caused by unrelated bacteria. The intoxicant bacterium *Staphylococcus aureus* causes staphylococcal toxic shock syndrome, and *Streptococcus pyogenes* causes the streptococcal form of the syndrome. Both produce a disease that starts out with a rapidly progressing fever, and that may lead to a drop in blood pressure, a decrease in kidney function, and a decline in liver performance. Shock can result in both diseases. People with staphylococcal toxic shock syndrome are more likely to have diarrhea, disorientation, muscle aches, nausea, and vomiting. These signs and symptoms reflect chemicals called superantigens, which overwork the immune system. Streptococcal toxic shock syndrome presents fewer signs and symptoms. However, it is a more severe disease than staphylococcal toxic shock syndrome because the bacteria are more aggressive in invading the body. *Streptococcus pyogenes* produces a variety of secretions that damage many body parts as well as tax the immune system.

Both of the organisms involved in toxic shock syndrome cause illness because they evade the host's natural defenses against disease. After all, these bacteria are common in healthy people. This means that the body is normally able to keep the bacteria in check. To cause disease, *Staphylococcus aureus* overwhelms the body's defenses by congregating large numbers of bacteria in one spot. It also is more likely to cause disease if other conditions or diseases weaken the immune system. *Streptococcus pyogenes* is a more aggressive organism than *Staphylococcus aureus.* It produces secretions that break down the barriers that normally protect against invasion by bacteria. However, *Streptococcus pyogenes* is more effective at causing disease if it gains entry into the body by breaches in the barriers. A weakened immune system also aids the bacterium.

3

Septic Diseases:
The Body Defends Itself

Nor ear can hear nor tongue can tell
The tortures of that inward hell.

George Gordon Byron, *The Giaour*

Lord Byron's passage from *The Giaour* could have portrayed septic diseases equally as well as it did Hell. A **septic disease**, or **sepsis**, refers to a painful condition involving the presence of microorganisms throughout the body. Normally, microorganisms do not inhabit the bloodstream and internal organs. However, this can occur when microorganisms bypass the body's defenses to invade the body and then spread to all the organ systems through the blood. Septic diseases are rarely mild. Even with treatment, they can lead to permanent bodily damage and death. Each organ system has its inventory of specific septic diseases. The most deadly septic diseases have to do with a total invasion of the body by microorganisms transported in the blood. These conditions include blood poisoning, or **septicemia**.

Bacteria, viruses, and fungi can cause septic diseases. Most of the septic disease microorganisms are normally pathogenic with a variety of characteristics that by design harm the body. Included in these characteristics are a host of secretions that digest body tissues, poison certain cells, and overstimulate the immune system. Many bacteria, numerous fungi, and all viruses intentionally produce disease in their attempts to survive in the body. However, not all microorganisms are harmful. Many live freely in the environment consuming decaying matter. Others inhabit the bodies of other organisms, coexisting without producing any harm. They usually feed on unwanted secretions on the skin or break down waste products in the digestive system. Many of these organisms provide a variety of benefits for their host organisms that they inhabit. However, under certain conditions, these safe microorganisms can accidentally cause **opportunistic diseases**. Illnesses that weaken the immune system can produce conditions in which harmless bacteria can invade the body to produce disease. Many septic conditions are due to rare situations whereby bacteria and fungi can freely enter the body and invade the organ systems.

The two types of bacteria that cause toxic shock syndrome normally produce similar diseases that can be distinguished only by careful medical examination. *Staphylococcus* bacteria most commonly cause skin infections. Some bacteria may enter the body and result in mild to severe wound infections (Figure 3.1). Others can enter the blood to produce immediate or long-term heart-valve diseases. *Streptococcus* bacteria are usually associated with respiratory infections, including "strep throat." They also cause earaches, wound infections, urinary tract diseases, and vaginal tract infections. Like *Staphylococcus*, *Streptococcus* can cause heart disease. Both of these bacteria are associated with mild cases of food poisoning. Toxic shock syndrome is a severe expression of a disease that has gotten out of control in the body. The bacteria seem to create an illusion of an infection that goes unchecked by the body. However, many signs and symptoms of toxic shock syndrome are due to the body's means of fighting off the infection.

Luckily, the body has a variety of defense mechanisms that reduce the chances of microorganisms causing disease. Even the most malicious microorganisms must put up a good battle against these body defenses before they can cause harm. There are two main categories of body defenses. One defense is **nonspecific immunity**, or **innate immunity**. It is composed of

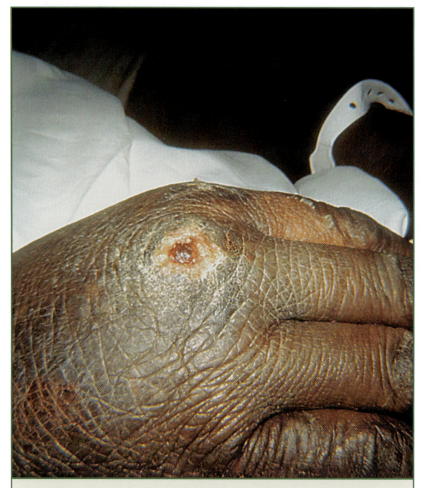

Figure 3.1 Wounds and a weakened immune system permit normally harmless bacteria and fungi to enter the body and invade organ systems. Bacteria which have entered the body can also cause wounds and eruptions on the skin

barriers which keep bacteria from invading the body. The other defense system is specific, or **acquired**, immunity. This type of immunity uses special cells to target a particular microorganism actively causing a disease. The nonspecific and specific immunities continuously work together to reduce the incidence of septic diseases. People with weaknesses in either of these defenses have increased probability and severity of disease by pathogens and opportunistic microorganisms.

NONSPECIFIC IMMUNITY

The first evidence of an organism's ability to fend off disease came from the research of Russian scientist Elie Metchnikoff in 1882 (Figure 3.2). His observations on young starfish showed how certain cells in the body responded to infection by devouring invading microorganisms. Scientists now know that the cells he discovered are part of an immune system response called nonspecific immunity. Nonspecific immunity uses general features of the body, such as skin and mucous membranes, to prevent the entrance or spread of infectious microorganisms. Skin and mucous membranes block micro-organisms by producing a virtual wall around the body. However, the cells recognized by Metchnikoff act differently. They kill pathogens with the same intent as a farmer spraying his crops to prevent against insects. Nonspecific immunity includes three types of defenses against infectious diseases: physical barriers, chemical deterrents, and **cellular** attack.

PHYSICAL BARRIERS

Mucous membranes and skin are the primary physical barriers designed to prevent invasion by microorganisms. They form a continuous layer of cells much like a brick wall surrounding the body and lining the **digestive tract** (Figure 3.3) and respiratory system. Their first function is to block invasion of the blood and internal organs by microorganisms. This barrier stops most microorganisms, and thus they can cause little or no harm to the body. However, some pathogenic microorganisms produce secretions that can break down the tight connections between cells, rendering the barrier useless until it heals or defends itself in other ways. Several of the microorganisms causing septic diseases have ways of breaching the barrier by

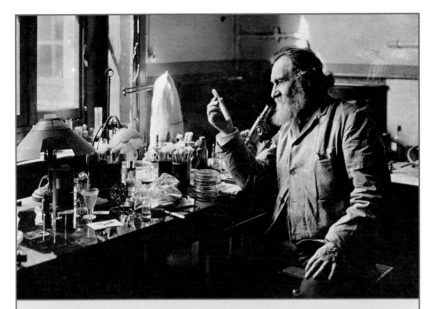

Figure 3.2 Elie Metchnikoff, shown here in his laboratory, was the first to recognize non-specific immunity in organisms. Metchnikoff was observing starfish and noticed how certain cells responded differently than normal cells to the invasion of microorganisms. These cells actually killed the invading microorganisms. Thus the idea of immune cells was born.

digesting or irritating the cells, permitting passage into under-lying tissues and the blood.

Mucus membranes help to trap microorganisms before they can enter the body and move them away from areas where they can potentially cause harm. For example, **mucus** secreted by the respiratory system's mucous membranes continuously moves upward from the lungs to throat. Once in the throat, the mucus makes its way to the digestive system, where it enters the harsh environment of the stomach. Along the way any microorganisms that may have entered the lungs or throat become stuck within the mucus. The digestive action of the stomach and intestines destroys the microorganisms along with the mucus. Almost all microorganisms will cling to the

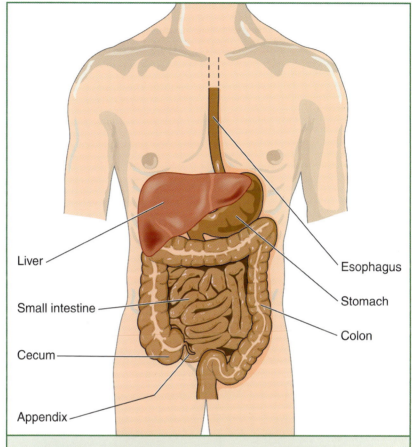

Liver

Small intestine

Cecum

Appendix

Esophagus

Stomach

Colon

Figure 3.3 As discussed in the chapter, mucous membranes line many body surfaces, including the digestive tract, shown here. Since the digestive tract provides a link to the outside environment, mucous membranes help to trap any foreign microorganisms that might harm the body. The digestive tract is one way that TSS organisms can enter the body.

mucus, making this a good system for clearing the lungs of disease. Unfortunately, air pollution and smoking reduce this action, making people more susceptible to diseases that invade the respiratory system.

Body secretions play a role in nonspecific immunity, acting as chemical barriers against infection. Sweat, for example, not only cools the body but also is important in prohibiting the growth of microorganisms on the skin. It possesses a slightly acidic chemistry that discourages the overgrowth of bacteria. After all, too much bacterial growth can encourage pathogens and induce harmless bacteria to irritate the skin, causing a breakdown in the physical barrier. The juices of the stomach are very acidic, which will kill any swallowed pathogens. Tears and urine also help ward off infectious diseases. They flush away microorganisms from the eyes and urinary tract, respectively. Moreover, they contain proteins called **enzymes** that discourage microbial growth. Lysosome, an enzyme found in tears and mucus, specifically attacks the types of bacteria that cause toxic shock syndrome. A group of enzymes called peroxidases found in body fluids and milk literally bleaches many microorganisms that make their way past the physical and chemical barriers on the body's surface.

Other chemical barriers circulating in the blood try to starve, poison, or break apart microorganisms. At least a dozen proteins secreted by blood cells mount a complex attack that helps with the removal of microbes that enter the body. They contribute to the fever, **inflammation**, and other signs associated with septic diseases such as toxic shock syndrome. Several proteins that make up the complement system of the blood bind to bacteria, ultimately producing openings in bacteria that cause them to die. Chemicals called interferons target viruses, leaving other microorganisms alone. Interferons prevent viruses from infecting body cells and help with the removal of cells already under viral attack.

A variety of immune system cells roaming the body and floating in the blood contribute to the nonspecific cellular attack component of the immune system. The nonspecific cells make many of the compounds produced for chemical protection of the body. In addition, many of the chemicals produced for the chemical defense stimulate the cellular attack. Large cells called **macrophages** circulate throughout the body, eating and destroying foreign material and uninvited microorganisms. They are very effective against many bacteria, but large invasions can easily overwhelm them. Macrophages inhabit body linings, preventing microorganisms from entering the body and the blood and tissues, attacking those that attempt to pass into the body. Cells called lymphocytes act as an early-warning system that alerts the body to microbial invasion. Many of the lymphocyte secretions stimulate the action of other immune-system cells. Some of the secretions directly fend off viruses. Cells called eosinophils and neutrophils assist with the early-warning system by signaling other cells about bacterial invasion. They also produce secretions that mount a chemical defense. Fever, as found in toxic shock syndrome, results from a group of cellular secretions called cytokines. Cytokines that specifically induce fever are called **pyrogens**, meaning to produce fire. Fever is not a negative consequence of disease but rather a method of killing septic bacteria. The elevated body temperatures produced during fever offset the metabolism of microorganisms, causing them to die off more readily. Fever works in combination with other defense mechanisms to starve bacteria and inhibit their reproduction.

SPECIFIC IMMUNITY

Specific immunity does its job by designing a specific attack catered to the microorganism causing the disease. It works to reduce the current invasion and provides a way for the body to react more readily to subsequent incursions. Specific immunity employs many of the components of nonspecific immunity, but it uses them in different ways, which results in the formation of a "memory" of a particular invasive microorganism. Unlike nonspecific immunity, specific immunity becomes stronger with increased exposure to the microorganism causing a disease and ensures quick resistance to further attacks. Several scientists working in England, France, and Germany discovered specific immunity concurrently. Included in this notable group of scientists was Louis Pasteur, who developed the process of pasteurization of milk and produced vaccines that stimulated specific immunity. The first person to recognize specific immunity was English physician Edward Jenner in 1796. He discovered that artificial triggering of specific immunity (such as through a vaccine) could protect the body from disease. Jenner noted this observation well before researchers understood the immune system and just as they were discovering microorganisms. His insight produced the technique called **variolation**, which doctors used to immunize people against **smallpox**.

Variolation involved introducing small amounts of a disease organism into the body of a healthy individual. As noted by physicians who practiced the technique, this action seemed to give people a mild form of the disease and protection from further infection by that particular microorganism. The technique exploited the body's two-stage means of protecting itself from repeated infection by disease organisms. In the

THE BIRTH AND NEAR-DEATH OF VACCINATION

Many physicians and almost all the public did not favorably receive Edward Jenner when he discovered variolation in 1796. Jenner treated his first patients by scratching or injecting them with animal body fluids. Superstitious beliefs at the time prevented people from believing that it was safe to be injected with animal body fluids. During that period of history people thought that blood contained the traits of an animal. Cells and genetic material were not discovered until much later. The common wisdom assumed that injecting people with animal body fluids introduces the animal's traits into the body. Rumors abounded of people developing cow-shaped growths and children born with cow parts. Luckily, the success of variolation overcame superstitious belief, paving the way for modern vaccination.

first stage, the same macrophages that carry out nonspecific immunity identify and destroy an invading microorganism. Upon identifying the microorganism, the macrophage then provides a memory of the particular offending microorganism. The second stage of specific immunity uses the memory developed in the first stage to mount an immediate attack against further encounters with the microorganism.

The first stage of specific immunity begins when a microorganism encounters a mucous membrane or enters the body by breaching the nonspecific defenses. Ultimately a macrophage comes upon the microorganism, if the immune system is working properly. Some researchers believe that alcohol, improper nutrition, persistent infections, smoking, and continuous stress reduce the macrophages' ability to contact the microorganism. The macrophage then engulfs and digests the microorganism. Digested components of the microorganism, called **antigens,** then appear on the surface of the macrophage. On its travels throughout the body, the macrophage next encounters specific immunity cells called lymphocytes that reside in **lymphatic tissue** (Figure 3.4). One type of lymphocyte, called the T-helper cell, attaches to the antigen on the surface of the macrophage. This alerts the T-helper cell that a particular microorganism identified by the antigen is in the body. The T-helper cell next binds to another lymphocyte called a B cell.

B cells produce protein secretions called antibodies. Antibodies are proteins that bind to particular antigens. B cells produce antibodies for almost any type of antigen that can enter the body. Proteins found on the surfaces of microorganisms and the cells of other organisms are easily recognized as antigens and generally produce a strong immune response. The T-helper cell selects a particular B cell that produces antibodies for the antigen appearing on the T cell surface. T-helper cell secretions called cytokines stimulate the B cells to divide rapidly in a process called clonal selection. The offspring

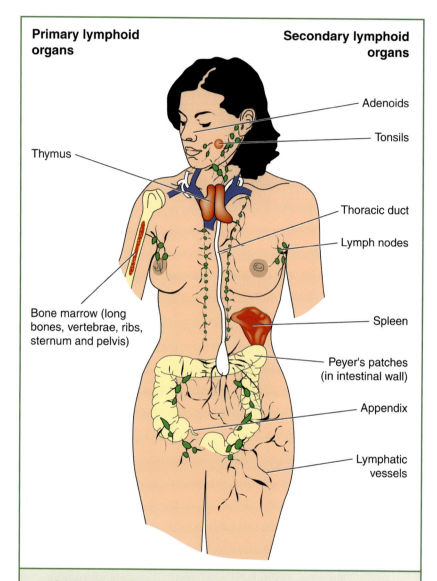

Primary lymphoid organs

Secondary lymphoid organs

Adenoids

Tonsils

Thymus

Thoracic duct

Lymph nodes

Bone marrow (long bones, vertebrae, ribs, sternum and pelvis)

Spleen

Peyer's patches (in intestinal wall)

Appendix

Lymphatic vessels

Figure 3.4 The immune system acts as the body's military, protecting it from harm by foreign microorganisms. The lymphatic system, illustrated here, is an important aspect of the immune system. Lymphocytes, special immune cells, originate from lymphatic tissue and can target, but specifically and non-specifically, different invading microorganisms such as the bacteria that cause TSS.

of the B cell, called plasma cells, then circulate around the body. The plasma cells carry a memory of a particular disease.

The immune system has "memory," meaning that once it has encountered a particular antigen, the next time that antigen is present the system is ready to produce large amounts of **antibodies**. Contact with the antibody causes B cells to release specific antibodies that attach to the antigen. By binding to antigens, antibodies are signaling to the body that an infection is taking place. This then starts a series of responses in which the body attempts to rapidly destroy and remove the antigen. Included in these responses is the activation of cells that can digest or poison microorganisms. Antibodies also make it easier for a lymphatic organ called the spleen to filter out microorganisms from the blood. This function of antibodies is crucial in combating septic diseases. Many septic diseases produce a large antibody response because most organisms causing the condition produce a wide array of antigens. This is especially true for the bacteria that cause toxic shock syndrome. They produce many antigens on their surfaces and many secretions recognized as antigens by the macrophages.

The second stage of immunity takes place when plasma cells encounter a microorganism that has previously caused disease. They immediately release antibodies upon contact with the microorganism. The rapid production of antibodies targets the microorganism for attack before it can further harm the body. These antibodies remain in place to protect the body if it is again infected by the same microorganism. Sometimes the body recognizes the microorganisms in the mucous membranes, before they can enter the rest of the body, thereby reducing the incidence of a severe infection. This plasma-cell response works best when a person regularly encounters the disease organism. Long periods between exposures to a disease tend to decrease the number of plasma cells that contribute to the memory of the disease. It usually takes about 5 to 10 years for the body to lose its memory of a disease. After that period, the body has to go through the first stage again to produce a new population of plasma cells for the disease organism. Illness, malnutrition, and stress reduce the second-stage response. This becomes very important when physicians try to predict why some people develop septic diseases more readily than others do.

MICROBIAL INVASION OF THE BODY

Even the most formidable body defenses cannot always keep bacteria from entering the body and causing disease. Organisms that cause septic diseases are a particular problem because they manage to evade the nonspecific immunity. This puts a greater burden on the specific immunity and may even lead to an excessive immune response. Too much activity by the immune system can cause the body to attack itself, creating a condition called **autoimmune disease**. Autoimmune disease is a typical outcome of septic diseases. The immune system can also fail to work if it is dealing with too many antigens at one time. This condition, called **immunosuppression**, makes it easier for septic disease organisms to spread around the body.

Septic diseases include a variety of conditions in which microorganisms invade deep within the body, usually traveling from the point of infection through the bloodstream. Most septic diseases start out when microorganisms which may be present on the skin under normal conditions unintentionally enter the blood or body tissues through wounds in the skin and mucous membranes, as is the case for toxic shock syndrome. An overpopulation of bacteria on mucous membranes can irritate the affected body part, causing bacteria to make their way into the body. A lack of personal hygiene and foreign objects placed in the body can produce conditions favorable for the overpopulation of bacteria. Even certain drug treatments may induce pathogenic bacteria to overgrow in response to a depletion of harmless bacteria. Harmless bacteria on the body compete with pathogens, preventing excessive growth of the pathogen. People with weakened immune systems are likely candidates for septic diseases as is shown with toxic shock syndrome. Finally, certain types of bacteria are naturally aggressive and readily breach the body's defenses, producing sepsis even in healthy people with fully functioning immune systems. Again, toxic shock syndrome can get its start this way. The septic disease called toxic shock syndrome confounds the immune system and the medical community by finding various avenues of causing disease.

4

Staphylococcus and STSS

The last phase and supreme goal of all human development is liberty.
Michael Bakunin, *Federalism, Socialism and Anti-Theologism*, 1867.

What does Bakunin's commentary regarding some people's refusal to seek liberty during the French revolution have to do with staphylococcal toxic shock syndrome? When confined by the body's defenses, *Staphylococcus* bacteria cause few, if any, problems for the body. At most, they can cause moderate skin irritation. On the other hand, when free to roam the body, this group of bacteria can cause a variety of severe problems, including toxic shock syndrome. *Staphylococcus* includes a variety of bacteria, many of which live in and on the bodies of animals. Most do not cause disease, whereas some are natural pathogens. Other *Staphylococcus* bacteria can cause disease as opportunistic pathogens, if things go wrong with the body's defenses or if the organism manages to overpopulate the body.

Researchers attributed the earliest recognized cases of toxic shock syndrome in the United States to *Staphylococcus* bacteria. Most occurrences today start out as a *Staphylococcus* infection that gets out of control. The fact that *Staphylococcus* bacteria occur in many places in the body and the environment makes it difficult to identify the sources of *Staphylococcus* infections. This also makes prevention difficult because the chance of encountering some type of *Staphylococcus* is very likely since it is found many places. *Staphylococcus* is present in food, in the soil, and on the skin and mouths of many organisms. The bacteria spread upon contact with objects and organisms and transfer themselves through water and air. In many cases, doctors cannot discover how the bacteria entered the body until they have thoroughly examined the patient. Physicians have to be cautious in speculating about the cause of a *Staphylococcus* infection, out of concern that they have missed the true origin. Even today, researchers scrutinize new cases of toxic shock syndrome to ensure that there are no new ways through which the disease is spreading.

THE *STAPHYLOCOCCUS* FAMILY

Microbiologists first identified *Staplylococcus* after the discovery of the microscope in the 1665. The bacteria were originally isolated from human skin and nasal cultures. Later, microbiologists used chemical tests and genetic analyses to categorize different types of *Staphylococcus*. Under the microscope, *Staphylococcus* looks like a group of spheres glued together in large clumps resembling bunches of grapes on a vine (Figure 4.1). These spherical cells are called **cocci**, (singular is coccus). There are many types of spherical bacteria, but only *Staphylococcus* bacteria grow in this characteristic clumping pattern. A covering called a **cell wall** surrounds the cell of *Staphylococcus*. Microbiologists classify the type of cell wall found on *Staphylococcus* as Gram-positive. Gram-positive describes the chemistry of a bacterium's cell wall based on a test called Gram staining (see box on page 51).

Scientists also can identify *Staphylococcus* by its method of obtaining food. *Staphylococcus* belongs to a group of bacteria called **facultative anaerobic chemoorganotrophs**. "Facultative anaerobic" means that *Staphylococcus* prefers oxygen, just as humans do, to carry out the life processes known as metabolism. However, the bacteria can live in the absence of oxygen if required. **Aerobic** bacteria must have oxygen to survive. "Chemoorganotroph" means that *Staphylococcus* must eat decaying organisms as food to obtain energy and raw materials to stay alive and reproduce. In its pursuit of food, *Staphylococcus*

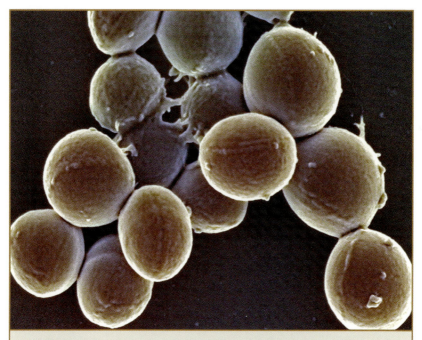

Figure 4.1 *Staphylococcus* bacteria are spherical in shape and usually clump together, looking like a bunch of grapes on a vine. An electron micrograph of *Staphylococcus* is shown here. The *Staphylococcus* group includes a variety of bacteria, many of which live in and on the bodies of animals, including humans.

produces a characteristic enzyme called catalase. Catalase protects *Staphylococcus* from harmful chemicals known as peroxides. The action of catalase is evident when you place hydrogen peroxide solution, available at grocery stores and pharmacies, on a wound or on your teeth. Catalase breaks down hydrogen peroxide into oxygen gas and water, producing a foaming mass of bubbles.

Knowing all this information about *Staphylococcus* helps scientists and physicians better understand the way *Staphylococcus* causes disease. This information also allows them to come up with effective methods for preventing and treating *Staphylococcus* diseases. For example, most Gram-positive bacteria produce exotoxins associated with disease. Exotoxins harm the body in various ways and help explain the signs and symptoms of a disease. Physicians have also learned that certain antibiotics are more effective against Gram-positive bacteria.

In addition to *Staphylococcus*, a host of other Gram-positive aerobic and facultative anaerobic chemoorganotrophic bacteria can be categorized into a larger group of bacteria called the *Micrococcaceae*. Other bacteria in this group include *Enterococcus*, *Micrococcus*, and *Streptococcus*. *Enterococcus* bacteria are a group of usually harmless bacteria that live in the intestines of many animals, including insects and mammals. Some types of *Enterococcus* bacteria can cause urinary tract infections and be spread as a sexually transmitted disease. *Micrococcus*

THE GRAM STAIN TECHNIQUE

Gram staining was named after Danish physician Hans Christian Joachim Gram who lived from 1853 to 1938. He developed the technique while looking for a quick way to identify bacteria in the lungs of people who died from pneumonia. In his investigation, he noticed that bacteria varied in their ability to absorb a stain or dye called crystal violet. Some bacteria remained stained purple when the specimens were washed with alcohol, while some did not. Unfortunately, the unstained bacteria could not be visualized under a microscope. Gram modified the staining technique by adding a pink dye called fuschin that remained in all the bacteria. Bacteria that retained the initial, purple stain (as can be seen in Figure 4.2) were considered Gram positive, such as *Staphylococcus*. Bacteria that lost the purple stain and appeared pink were designated Gram negative. Gram stain properties tell much about the way these bacteria cause disease. Gram positive bacteria are very likely to secrete toxins that create many of the symptoms of disease. Whereas, Gram negative bacteria mostly produce disease by activities other than secreting toxins.

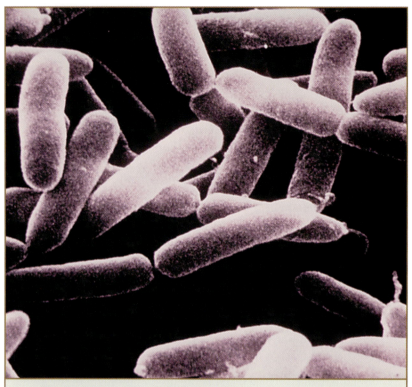

Figure 4.2 Current genetic studies show that *Staphylococcus* bacteria are closely related to rectangular-shaped, gram-positive bacterial known as *Bacillus* (shown here) and *Lactobacillus*.

bacteria occur everywhere, even on dust particles in seemingly clean environments. We know little about its ability to cause significant disease. The *Streptococcus* group, like *Staphylococcus*, includes common bacteria known to cause mild to severe disease. *Streptococcus* will be discussed further in the next chapter. Of all the forms of *Micrococcaceae*, most physicians would agree that *Staphylococcus* bacteria are clinically the most important because they cause the most disease. The fact that these are common bacteria make it likely that people will come across a situation in which *Staphylococcus* will cause a disease, and thus must be more aware of these types of bacteria. Physicians put much effort into combating ailments caused by *Staphylococcus.*

TYPES OF *STAPHYLOCOCCUS*

The most recent analysis of bacterial classification, reported in the 1992 edition of *Bergey's Manual of Systematic Bacteriology*, identified 19 types of *Staphylococcus.* Scientists knew of only two types in 1884. Science has come a long way in isolating and identifying microorganisms since 1884. One bacterium was named *Staphylococcus aureus* (refer again to Figure 4.1) because of its yellow appearance. *Aureus* comes from the Latin word for gold. The other type of bacteria they named *Staphylococcus albus* because it formed a white growth when raised in laboratory cultures. *Albus* is from the Latin word for a bright-white reflection or dawn light. *Staphylococcus albus* was not one, but a group of *Staphylococcus* species. The orginal *Staphylococcus albus* was believed to be a specimen of *Staphylococcus epidermidis.* Current genetic studies have shown that the *Staphylococcus* bacterium is a closer relative to rectangular-shaped Gram-positive bacteria known as *Bacillus* and *Lactobacillus. Bacillus* (Figure 4.2) and *Lactobacillus* are not included in the *Micrococcaceae.* The deadly biological warfare bacterium, anthrax, is also a type of *Bacillus. Lactobacillus* includes harmless bacteria found in milk. They produce the characteristic sour taste to cheese and yogurt.

Scientists currently divide *Staphylococcus* into two groups: the aureus and non-aureus bacteria. The aureus group comprises only the various strains of *Staphylococcus aureus* noted in 1884. There are many types of non-aureus *Staphylococcus*, with *Staphylococcus epidermidis* representing the most medically important type. The *Staphylococcus epidermidis* group includes *Staphylococcus auricularis*, found growing on the outer parts of the human ear, and *Staphylococcus capitis*, an inhabitant of human skin like *Staphylococcus epidermidis.* Both lack the secretions that would make them highly pathogenic, and no ailments have been associated with these *Staphylococcus* bacteria. Scientists have collected a pathogenic bacterium, called *Staphylococcus hominis*, from human blood cultures. This *Staphylococcus* is very dangerous because common antibiotics do not readily kill it.

Many common food products contain *Staphylococcus* bacteria. Tofu and soy-sauce lovers may not wish to know that *Staphylococcus carnosus* and *Staphylococcus condimenti* occur in the soy mash used to make these foods. **Fermented** fish products typical of Asian cuisine contain the harmless *Staphylococcus piscifermentans*. Other *Staphylococcus* bacteria found in foods are *Staphylococcus caseilyticus* and *Staphylococcus fleurettii*, which break down the proteins in milk products. Others in the non-aureus group are *Staphylococcus arlettae*, *Staphylococcus caprae*, and *Staphylococcus gallinarum*, found in domesticated and wild animals. None of these cause human ailments. *Staphylococcus delphini* of dolphins, *Staphylococcus sciuri* of rodents, and *Staphylococcus lutrae* of otters have the ability to cause human disease, just as they do in the respective animals. People who hunt these animals for food and fur can contract mild to severe infections. Pets also carry *Staphylococcus* that may cause human disease. *Staphylococcus equaroum* in various pets, *Staphylococcus schleiferi* in dogs, and *Staphylococcus felis,* limited to cats, have been isolated from diseased animals.

Knowledge of the different types of *Staphylococcus* is critical for understanding how these bacteria cause problems for humans. Scientists investigate the properties of the various *Staphylococci* to find common characteristics that make one harmless or make another pathogenic. It is also important to know why some are harmless in one organism but cause disease in others. Most important is that this knowledge gives a better understanding of the *Staphylococcus* bacterium that causes toxic shock syndrome and other human disorders.

THE TOXIC SHOCK SYNDROME *STAPHYLOCOCCUS*

The cause of Staphylococcal Toxic Shock Syndrome, or STSS, is a particularly pathogenic *Staphylococcus* bacterium called *Staphylococcus aureus*. It appears to be specific to humans and unrelated to other *Staphylococcus* bacteria. The CDC recently called *Staphylococcus aureus* an emerging "superbug" because of its potential to cause a scourge of severe, incurable diseases. *Staphylococcus aureus* is a pathogen because of its ability to breach the body's immune defense mechanisms. It does this with a variety of enzymes that permit the bacterium to eat a diet of decaying animals. Unfortunately, the same enzymes contribute to its ability to digest living animals. *Staphylococcus aureus* also has a collection of chemicals that protect it from the body defenses that would kill other micro-organisms. Many of these protective measures developed so the bacterium can coexist on the human body safely. This is normally not dangerous to an organism unless the bacterium is causing disease.

Staphylococcus aureus carries an arsenal of assorted chemicals and enzymes that contribute to human disease. One characteristic chemical called **coagulase** stimulates blood clotting. Scientists believe that coagulase protects bacteria from attack by the body's white blood cells. Blood clots that form around the bacteria provide a protective barrier that prevents white blood cells from making contact. White blood cells cannot assist with the removal and destruction of bacteria if they cannot access the bacterial cells. An enzyme called staphylokinase also aids clotting. It ensures that the clots remain intact as long as the bacteria are active. Leukocidins are another group of chemical toxins that impair white blood cells. These chemicals kill any white blood cell that encounters *Staphylococcus aureus*. This strategy is very effective in inhibiting macrophages that alert the immune system to a bacterial invasion. Leukocidins work by poking holes in the white blood cells. This blocking and loss of white blood cells explains why *Staphylococcus aureus* can spread unimpeded throughout the body. It also explains how large populations of *Staphylococcus aureus* can overgrow the mucous membranes and skin without detection.

The cell wall of *Staphylococcus aureus* contains components that prevent destruction by the immune system without harming white blood cells. The cell wall is also loaded with a complex chemical called peptidoglycan, a combination sugar-protein substance that permits all Gram-positive bacteria (Figure 4.3) to attach tightly to the mucous membranes and skin. This makes it difficult for the body to remove the bacteria, and the bacteria remain securely concealed in safe places away from the immune system. A related chemical called capsular polysaccharide forms an indigestible layer covering the cell wall. This chemical prevents digestion of *Staphylococcus aureus* by white blood cells called macrophages that normally eat and destroy microbial invaders. The capsular polysaccharide disables macrophages but does not destroy them. A protein called *protein A* also keeps the bacterium from digestion by macrophages. Protein A blocks antibodies that would normally bind to the surface of *Staphylococcus aureus.* Since macrophages seek out bacteria labeled with antibodies, *Staphylococcus aureus* evades the immune system by hiding from the antibodies. Thus the body has a difficult time locating and removing *Staphylococcus aureus* once it has spread throughout the body.

Staphylococcus aureus also secretes digestive enzymes that turn animal tissues into food suitable for bacteria. One characteristic enzyme of *Staphylococcus aureus* is hemolysin. Hemolysin means to "break red blood cells." As its name implies, the enzyme degrades red blood cells that are essential for carrying oxygen in the blood. This condition contributes to an anemia-like condition that makes the victim easily fatigued. In severe infections, the destruction of red blood cells can greatly exceed the body's ability to replace the cells. The spleen, located below the stomach, is able to store approximately one

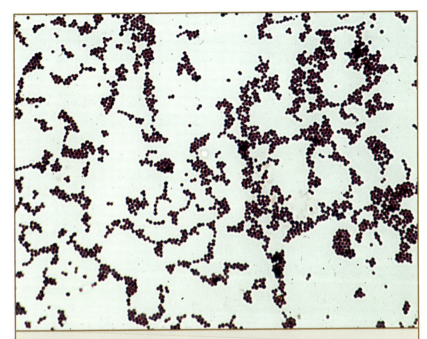

Figure 4.3 Gram-positive bacteria stain purple, such as the *Bacillus subtilus* shown in this picture. Gram-positive bacteria retain the crystal violet-iodine stain due to special properties of their cell walls.

pint of red blood cells for quick release. However, the body produces new red blood cells at a slow rate. Diseases such as toxic shock syndrome make the condition worse by slowing down red-blood-cell replacement.

Other digestive enzymes include deoxyribonuclease, hyaluronidase, and lipase. Deoxyribonuclease, also known as DNase, digests the DNA or genetic material of killed cells. Fast-growing bacteria such as *Staphylococcus aureus* need large amounts of digested DNA to keep up their high rate of reproduction. Again, this explains the great success of *Staphylococcus aureus* as it spreads throughout the afflicted individual. Hyaluronidase is an enzyme that degrades an important cell "glue" called hyaluronic acid. Hyaluronic acid holds much of the body together acting like a skeleton that holds cells in place. Thus, the enzyme not only provides *Staphylococcus aureus* with food, it also makes it easier for the bacterium to invade new parts of the body because when it breaks down, it allows access to the blood and tissues. Lipase breaks down the fats that make up a large component of animal cells. This permits *Staphylococcus aureus* to kill and digest cells it needs for food. Fat is essential for rapid bacterial growth. The lipase may also help *Staphylococcus aureus* disable immune-system cells that attack bacteria. A horrible consequence of lipase secretion is that it sometimes results in the disfiguring destruction of the fatty tissues underlying the skin. Hyaluronidase and lipase in large amounts can lead to a condition in which the bacteria appear to eat the flesh from underneath the skin.

Exfoliatins are a group of enzyme-like chemicals that give toxic shock syndrome its characteristic sign of reddened and peeling flesh. The chemicals break down the connections between skin cells, making them shed more easily. Small amounts of exfoliatins on the mucous membranes and skin lead to redness and irritations. However, large levels of exfoliatins will cause severe peeling of the skin, giving the impression that the skin was burned. This is the "scalded skin" appearance that shows up regularly in advanced cases of toxic shock syndrome. Proteases are another group of enzymes that specifically degrade skin. However, some can digest a protein collagen that provides the shape and structure for other tissues. They digest the protein connections holding cells together and aid in the degradation of dead cells. Exfoliatins and proteases, working together with hyaluronidase and lipase, can contribute to disfigurement of the skin.

The last group of chemicals that make *Staphylococcus aureus* a pathogen is the enterotoxins. This potent group of chemicals was discussed in Chapter 2. Recall that they poison the immune system cells and contribute to the fever, headache, nausea, and pain associated with toxic shock syndrome.

Included in the group of enterotoxins produced by *Staphylococcus aureus* are Enterotoxins A, B, C, C2, D, E, and F. TSST is another enterotoxin that contributes to cell damage and other signs and symptoms. Luckily, the body uses enterotoxins as antigens to signal that microorganisms are present in the body. Then the body can carry out an immune attack as long as the enterotoxins are present. Sometimes the enterotoxins persist after the bacteria are dead, ensuring that the body is primed to prevent an immediate recurrence of the disease.

Not all *Staphylococcus aureus* bacteria produce the same types and quantities of enzymes and toxins. The degree and nature of the secretions determine the severity of infection. Scientists identify different strains of *Staphylococcus aureus* by the combination of secretions they produce. For example, those that secrete only two or three enterotoxins produce a milder reaction than bacteria that release several of the toxins. Less invasive *Staphylococcus aureus* are deficient in the amounts of enzymes they secrete. Consequently, they cannot spread rapidly and readily throughout the body. This variation means that adequate diagnosis and treatment requires knowledge of the strain causing toxic shock syndrome. The diagnosis is taught in medical school, but many doctors see so few cases that it becomes difficult to recognize. Physicians must collect samples of *Staphylococcus aureus* for thorough analysis in a medical laboratory. One particular variation is confounding efforts to treat and prevent toxic shock syndrome.

Some strains of *Staphylococcus aureus* produce proteins that protect them from treatment with antibiotics. One enzyme, called beta lactamase (also known as penicillinase), makes the bacterium invulnerable to the common antibiotic penicillin. Bacteria that are resistant to antibiotics are termed "superbugs." These bacteria are difficult if not impossible to treat according to conventional strategies of controlling microorganisms.

5

Streptococcus and StrepTSS

The instinct to command others, in its primitive essence, is a carnivorous, altogether bestial and savage instinct.

Michael Bakunin, *Protestation of the Alliance*, 1871.

The fearsome instinct to dominate others mentioned by Bakunin described the tendencies of people in ruling positions throughout human history. This account equally describes *Streptococcus* bacteria. Most of these bacteria are capable of doing harm to animals and plants that they happen to encounter. Almost all *Streptococcus* bacteria carry traits that give them the ability to cause disease. They are more likely to cause disease than the *Staphylococcus* bacteria mentioned in Chapter 4. All occur in association with animals carrying out some function that does not always lead to harm. When the opportunity arises, however, almost all *Streptococcus* bacteria have features that unleash conditions ranging from mild discomfort to excruciating, fatal disease.

Certain cases of toxic shock syndrome could not be linked to *Staphylococcus* infections. Researchers discovered that these cases of toxic shock syndrome could be attributed to *Streptococcus*. Toxic shock syndrome caused by *Streptococcus* has the abbreviation StrepTSS to distinguish it from staphylococcal toxic shock syndrome, or STSS. StrepTSS produces a similar set of conditions to STSS. However, there are significant differences in the degree of signs and symptoms. Differences in the types of enzymes and toxins secreted produce these variations. A comprehensive blood examination is usually necessary to confirm the bacterium causing the toxic shock syndrome is present in the patient's body. Scientists identified StrepTSS in the late 1980s, almost 10 years after confirmation of STSS. This finding initially upset many physicians because they may have inadvertently diagnosed cases of StrepTSS as STSS. This new disease added another complication to their vigilance against toxic shock syndrome.

THE *STREPTOCOCCUS* FAMILY

Scientists knew the actions of *Streptococcus* bacteria and their relatives well before bacteria were discovered. Various types of *Streptococcus* were involved in common human disorders ranging from sore throats to wound infections without physicians knowing that these conditions were caused by one type of bacterium. Many of the adverse effects of *Streptococcus* infections appear in war records dating back 3000 years. However, the people of the time had other explanations for the infections, none of which pertained to infectious microorganisms. Bacteria related to *Streptococcus* were also used in the process of fermentation, unsuspectingly being cultivated more than 10,000 years ago to produce fermented beverages and foods. It was not until the perfection of the microscope in 1665 that the possibility of microscopic life arose. Unbeknownst to Dutch scientist Antony van Leeuwenhoek, he observed and drew bacteria while studying different specimens under his newly developed microscope. It took another 100 years before scientists identified and named bacteria and showed them to be the cause of disease and **fermentation**. It was Anton Julius Friedrich Rosenbach, who also named *Staphylococcus*, who named *Streptococcus* in 1884.

Streptococcus is traditionally lumped with *Staphylococcus* as Gram-positive chemoorganotrophic bacteria. As mentioned earlier, Gram-positive bacteria stain purple with the dye crystal violet and are likely to produce secreted toxins. Similar to *Staphylococcus*, *Streptococcus* cells have a sphereical shape and are also called cocci. However, the cells of *Streptococcus* organize themselves into straight chains of varying lengths instead of the branching chains of *Staphylococcus*. The term "strepto" in its name refers to the twisted appearance of the chains. These simple-to-culture bacteria prefer anaerobic growth, but they can tolerate oxygenated enviroments unlike many other anaerobic bacteria. Oxygen is usually toxic to strict anaerobic bacteria. This feature makes it possible for *Streptococcus* to survive in a variety of environments. Its ability to live on aerobic surfaces of the skin as well as the anaerobic conditions of the digestive system is evidence of this bacterium's versatility at surviving. Luckily, it is sensitive to chemicals and conditions normally used to clean surfaces of microbial growth.

The closest relative of *Streptococcus* is a type of bacterium called *Enterococcus*. The two are sometimes categorized together as the *Streptococcus/Enterococcus* group, noted for lacking the enzyme catalase normally produced by *Staphylococcus*. Thus, these bacteria do not show the characteristic bubbling test when exposed to hydrogen peroxide. They are also missing an enzyme called oxidase that is involved in aerobic respiration. This means that *Streptococcus* survive better in the absence of oxygen. *Streptococcus* and *Enterococcus* cannot use oxygen to carry out living processes as they break down food. Consequently, this characteristic results in the production of a multitude of waste products that can cause ailments on their own or can aggravate a disease due to other activities of the bacteria. *Enterococcus faecalis* (Figure 5.1), the most notable of these bacteria, is usually not pathogenic and normally lives in the digestive system of animals. It will sometimes cause urinary tract infections and sexually transmitted diseases. Sometimes *Enterococcus* can create problems if it invades a body with a severely damaged digestive system. It harms the body by secreting enzymes that break down internal organs. Other related bacteria include *Aerococcus*, an opportunistic pathogen; *Lactococcus*, which invades wounds; *Leuconostoc*, reported to cause septicemia; and *Pediococcus*, also known to cause sepsis.

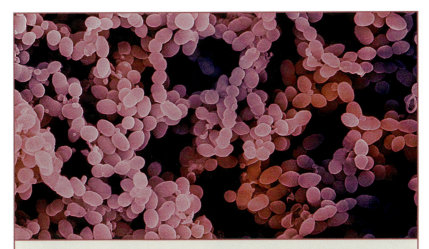

Figure 5.1 Certain bacteria related to *Streptococcus* are not harmful and are normally found living on or in humans and animals. *Enterococcus faecalis* (shown here) is a close relative to *Streptococcus* and normally lives in the digestive system of animals. Although it is normally harmless, it can occasionally cause urinary tract infections and sexually transmitted diseases.

Streptococcus, as is true for all Gram-positive bacteria, secrete a variety of toxins, called exotoxins, that can cause mild to severe damage to the body. They also contain a protective capsule similar to the one found on *Staphylococcus*, which protects the bacterium from certain environmental conditions and body defenses. *Streptococcus* bacteria are medically important because many of them produce enzymes and toxins that cause disease. Bacteria such as *Streptococcus* that are proficient at resisting immune system defenses probably have a long history of harming their animal hosts. Over the generations, these bacteria adapted defenses to ensure their survival in a host. Some *Streptococcus* started out as innocuous inhabitants of humans and accidentally picked up pathogenic characteristics. Others became harmful only if they got into parts of the body where they did not belong or if their population rose as the result of other diseases. Then there are *Streptococcus* bacteria found naturally on one animal that accidentally cause disease in other animals. These bacteria usually create no problems for their natural host. However, on the wrong host they pose a threat.

TYPES OF *STREPTOCOCCUS*

All *Streptococcus* bacteria look alike under the microscope. They are also hard to distinguish in microbiological cultures. Thus, it is almost impossible to tell them apart by looking at them, and instead, metabolic tests must be used to distinguish the various bacteria of the *Streptococcus* group. This is unlike the two groups of *Staphylococcus*, which have different colors in culture. Scientists believe that there are at least 40 confirmed types of *Streptococcus*, each having a few different strains. Scientists divide the 40 or more different types into 2 groups called **clusters**. Initially, the degree of **hemolysins** produced by the bacteria defined the clusters. Some *Streptococcus* do not produce any hemolysins and thus are nonhemolytic. Others produce either alpha or beta **hemolysis**. A beta-hemolytic *Streptococcus* produces the most severe effects in the body. A later method, called Lancefield grouping, categorized the types of *Streptococcus* based on immunological testing called **serotyping**. A particular Lancefield group refers to a protein antigen found on the surface of the bacteria. A combination of characteristics, including where the bacteria appear, presently determines the clusters. The clusters are the anginosus group, the bovis group, the mitis group, the mutans group, the **pyogenic** group, and the salivarius group.

 Streptococcus anginosus and a host of relatives make up the anginosus group. These alpha-hemolytic bacteria are common inhabitants of the mouth and nose and do not cause disease. They are part of the A, F, and G Lancefield groups The bovis group consists of an intestinal bacterium called *Streptococcus bovis*. As its name implies, scientists isolated it from the intestinal tract of cattle. These *Streptococci* are alpha- or nonhemolytic and related to other *Streptococcus* bacteria specific to particular animals. Most cause no harm in their host animals. However, they can infect wounds and cause septic diseases. They have a D Lancefield grouping. The mitis group contains a diversity of alpha-hemolytic bacteria in the H and O Lancefield groups. Most live in the respiratory systems of humans and animals without causing disease. These bacteria can cause some types of pneumonia. *Streptococcus pneumoniae*, which causes human respiratory diseases, is a pathogen in the mitis group. The mutans group has no hemolysins and does not belong to a designated Lancefield group. They live in the mouths of many animals, where they glue themselves to the teeth. Many of them are involved in tooth decay and possibly gum disease. *Streptococcus salivarius* appropriately appears in the salivarius group. Like the mutans-group bacteria, they live in the mouth and do not produce hemolysin. They belong to the K Lancefield group.

The pyogenes group contains the bacterium that causes StrepTSS. These bacteria are beta-hemolytic and are highly capable of causing severe reactions. They are part of the A, B, and C Lancefield groups. Included in the pyogenes group are *Streptococcus algalactiae*, *Streptococcus equisimilis*, and *Streptococcus pyogenes*.

Streptococcus algalactiae is a **contagious** bacterium of mammals. It commonly causes ear, sinus, and throat infections of domesticated animals and humans. People who work with animals are likely to contract infections from this bacterium. In the 1960s, *Streptococcus algalactiae* became a leading cause of disease in human babies.

Streptococcus equisimilis has several strains found in many mammals. They cause diseases similar to toxic shock syndrome in animals and humans. The bacteria spread thoughout the body causing high fever and damage to internal organs.

Streptococcus pyogenes is the culprit that produces StrepTSS and other diseases in humans. Researchers also called it *Streptococcus hemolyticus*, *Streptococcus erysipelatos*, *Streptococcus scarlatinae*, and *Micrococcus scarlatinae* until they confirmed that all were the same bacterium. Their small size and the high variability of traits make bacteria difficult to identify.

THE TOXIC SHOCK SYNDROME *STREPTOCOCCUS*

Streptococcus pyogenes is one of the most common pathogenic bacteria of humans. This particular type of *Streptococcus* is most often associated with diseases in humans. Other animals may harbor the bacterium in their bodies, but whether it causes disease in these animals is unknown. Like *Staphylococcus, Streptococcus* has many characteristics that produce illness in its host. In contrast to *Staphylococcus, Streptococcus pyogenes* is a more aggressive pathogen that can cause disease under normal conditions in healthy people. *Streptococcus pyogenes* primarily inhabits the skin and respiratory system. It is not found in the digestive system like other types of *Streptococcus.* Thus, it can only enter the body through a few very specific routes.

Natural pathogens such as *Streptococcus pyogenes* have features called **virulence factors** that enable them to cause disease. These factors provide a variety of characteristics that permit the bacterium to reside in the host and evade the host's immune system and are similar to the disease-causing characteristics of *Staphylococcus* mentioned in Chapter 4. Some examples of virulence factors include the cell wall and cellular secretions. The secretions include antigens, enzymes, and toxins that assist with various functions needed to feed and fend off the host's immune defenses. These defenses also give *Streptococcus pyogenes* its name. The word "pyogenes" comes from the Greek term "pyogenic," meaning to produce **pus**. Pus is an indication of severe disease. It contains a large concentration of white blood cells, immune-system fluids, and bacteria. Do not confuse pyogens with pyrogens. Pyrogens, a term derived from the Greek word *burn* which means producing fire or warmth, are chemicals that create a fever.

Streptococcus pyogenes gains a foothold in the body by using cell wall proteins called **adhesins**. Adhesins help microbes stick to the cells of other organisms. These adhesive proteins are not the same as the proteins that are normal constituents of the Gram-positive cell wall. Adhesions are solely for the purpose of attaching the bacterium to host tissues. As mentioned in Chapter 4, *Staphylococcus* adheres to its host using sticky components naturally found in the cell wall. *Streptococcus pyogenes* possesses a special adhesin called F protein. F protein ensures that *Streptococcus pyogenes* will bind to host proteins in a way that permits the bacterium to slip easily between the cells of the body. This enables *Streptococcus pyogenes* to pass through the mucous membranes and skin without the need for an opening. *Staphylococcus* and other bacteria usually gain entry into the body through damaged portions of the mucous membranes and skin. Another adhesin called M protein makes *Streptococcus pyogenes* difficult to remove from the mucous membranes and skin. M protein sticks specifically to the cells of these tissues. Scientists use M protein to detect different types of *Streptococcus*. Scientists have identified 80 different types of M proteins in bacteria.

Other cell wall components also protect *Streptococcus pyogenes* from destruction by the body's immune defenses. M protein not only allows the bacterium to stick to cells but it also inhibits digestion by macrophages. Another protein called M-like protein protects *Streptococcus pyogenes* in a similar manner. M-like proteins also cloak the bacterium from the host's immune system. *Streptococcus pyogenes* uses the M-like proteins to glue host proteins to its surface, making the body think the bacterium is a body cell. A capsule covers the cell wall of *Streptococcus pyogenes*, protecting it from digestion by macrophages. The capsule may resemble a body component of animals called hyaluronic acid. Thus, the body is less likely to attack *Streptococcus pyogenes* because it is tricked into treating the bacterium as a normal part of the body. Another protein called C5a peptidase permits *Streptococcus pyogenes* to avoid immune-system chemicals called complements. **Complements** label invading microbes for destruction and removal by the immune system (Figure 5.2).

Streptococcus pyogenes, like other Gram-positive bacteria, produce secretions that confound the body's immune response. On the top of the list is a potent group of poisons called exotoxins. *Streptococcus pyogenes* secrete various pyrogenic exotoxins that induce fever in the host. Scientists call these pyrogens *Streptococcus pyogenes* exotoxins, which they abbreviate as SPE A, SPE B, and SPE C. These exotoxins can cause immediate death when laboratory animals receive an injection of small amounts. SPE A is usually associated with killing the organism outright, whereas SPE B induces specific death to the heart muscle cells. All three of these exotoxins will produce a rash on the mucous membranes and skin (Figure 5.3). Chemicals that produce a rash are called erythrogenic toxins. Erythrogen means to turn something red. Scientists now know that different strains of *Streptococcus pyogenes* produce varying amounts of the pyrogens, making some strains more dangerous. Aside from producing fever, pyrogens overstimulate the immune system. This then causes the body to destroy itself accidentally, producing an abnormal condition called autoimmunity. Much of the tissue decay of StrepTSS is due to the body unintentionally destroying itself. This condition is very difficult to treat and any treatments could encourage further spread of *Streptococcus pyogenes*.

A variety of enzymes that destroy host cells and tissues occur in all strains of *Streptococcus pyogenes*. Hemolysins, similar to ones produced by *Staphylococcus*, destroy red blood cells, making available a rich supply of iron and protein needed for rapid bacterial growth. Streptolysin O and S are two hemolysins unique to *Streptococcus pyogenes*. Injections of these enzymes cause immediate death to laboratory animals. The enzyme hyaluronidase helps *Streptococcus pyogenes* digest their way through the body, permitting them to invade any tissue readily. The body secretes deoxyribonuclease, or DNase,

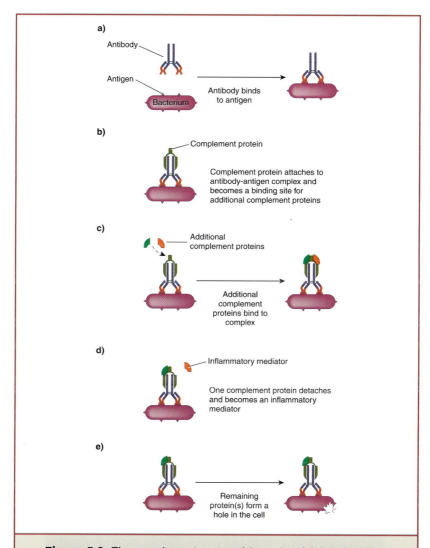

a)

Antibody

Antigen

Bacterium

Antibody binds to antigen

b)

Complement protein

Complement protein attaches to antibody-antigen complex and becomes a binding site for additional complement proteins

c)

Additional complement proteins

Additional complement proteins bind to complex

d)

Inflammatory mediator

One complement protein detaches and becomes an inflammatory mediator

e)

Remaining protein(s) form a hole in the cell

Figure 5.2 The complement system (shown here) labels invading microorganisms for destruction. An antibody binds to the antigen (foreign cell). A complement protein binds to the antibody and then breaks apart. One part of the complement protein remains attached to the antibody and serves to attract other complement proteins. The other fragment detaches from the antibody and searches out other complement proteins. Eventually, many complement proteins will attach to a cell and cause it to burst.

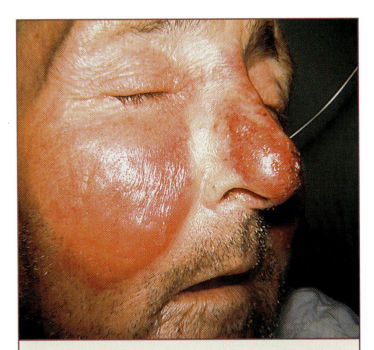

Figure 5.3 *Streptococcus pyogenes* secretions called pyogenes produce the characteristic skin rash of StrepTSS. These secretions contain exotoxins, which can be deadly if they occur in large amounts. One of the first signs that these exotoxins are present is the red rash, seen here on this man.

to assist with the digestion of DNA from dying cells. This provides *Streptococcus pyogenes* with the nutrients needed for rapid reproduction. *Streptococcus pyogenes* produces two unique enzymes called lipoproteinase and streptokinase. The role of lipoproteinase is unknown. However, most production occurs in strains of *Streptococcus pyogenes* that cause skin infections. The strain of *Streptococcus pyogenes* identified to cause StrepTSS does not secrete large amounts of this enzyme. Streptokinase plays a unique role by breaking down blood clots. This prevents *Streptococcus pyogenes* from being barricaded by blood clots that would restrict its movement throughout the body. This function is assisted by a cell-wall component called plasminogen-binding site protein. *Staphylococcus* does the opposite by encouraging clots that hide it from the immune system. *Streptococcus pyogenes* does not need that type of protection from the body.

The different severities of disease caused by *Streptococcus pyogenes* relate directly to the combination of features found in a particular strain of the bacterium. This makes it challenging for physicians who have to diagnose diseases caused by *Streptococcus pyogenes.* The bacteria found in blood samples must be thoroughly tested to determine the type of damage they can produce. The tests also permit the physician to predict the outcome of the disease. It helps to know whether the bacteria are going to stay on the mucous membranes or are likely to invade the whole body. Physicians also need to know how good the bacteria are at evading the host's immune system.

SAVING LIVES WITH BACTERIAL TOXINS

The same toxins that bring about the signs and symptoms of toxic shock have beneficial value if used in creative ways. The enzyme streptokinase secreted by *Streptococcus* normally helps the bacterium by preventing clot formation in its host. The inability to form clots permits the bacteria better access to the blood and body organs. However, as a medicine, streptokinase can break down blood clots that complicate heart disease. Physicians learned that streptokinase could be injected into the blood in low dosages without harming people. These injections are therapeutic in people who form blood clots that block important blood vessels of the heart and brain. A host of other bacterial secretions are being employed for diverse medical uses such as helping skin to heal without a scar to selectively killing cancer cells without harming the rest of the body.

6

Epidemiology of Toxic Shock Syndrome

There is properly no history, only biography.
Ralph Waldo Emerson (1803–1882), essayist

Epidemiology is the study of the history and transmission of a disease. Disease histories usually appear as biographies of people with the disease. Emerson would have been right on target if he were explaining the epidemiology of toxic shock syndrome. The best description of this disease is an accumulation of stories about afflicted individuals. A complete account of these people is essential to understand why they were suffering from toxic shock syndrome. Every action and each little habit require investigation for a full understanding of disease transmission. This can become particularly embarrassing when the disease spreads through sexual contact or inadequate personal hygiene. The latter of these disease factors was part of the reason for the occurrence of toxic shock syndrome. Complicating the investigation of toxic shock syndrome is the fact that several types of bacteria can cause the disease in different ways.

The Centers for Disease Control and Prevention (CDC) in Atlanta, Georgia, is the central location for epidemiological studies in the United States. It works together with other nations to build an international database of infectious diseases. With this information, researchers can predict the potential for a disease to spread worldwide. Public health agencies and physicians regularly report incidents of disease to the CDC. Doctors must report many diseases, including toxic shock syndrome, on special forms supplied by the agency. They use forms CDC 52.3, Toxic-Shock Syndrome Case Report and DCH-0952, Streptococcus (Group A) Invasive Disease form, to give accounts of toxic shock syndrome. The advent of the Internet makes this an easier task because forms can be downloaded from the CDC and submitted electronically through special Web access. This information is available to the public online or through a publication called the *Morbidity and Mortality Weekly Report.* Morbidity means illness and mortality means death. Pamphlets also provide information for every major disease. News alerts, pamphlets, and press releases report new occurrences of toxic shock syndrome, just after confirmation.

Scientists who study epidemiology are known as epidemiologists. They must use precise terms to describe the spread of disease to avoid confusion and misinterpretation of their findings. A typical epidemiological study begins with data collection.

TRACKING DISEASE WITH THE CDC

The Centers for Disease Control and Prevention (CDC) in Atlanta, Georgia, is a large research facility next to the Emory University Campus. It is a division of a massive agency called the United States Department of Health and Human Services (HHS). Most people are familiar with its work on infectious diseases. News stories about diseases such as SARS and monkey pox always contain comments from CDC scientists. Plus, the CDC is the first agency to distribute public information about diseases raising concerns in the news. The CDC is also the first place public health officials call with concerns about unfamiliar illnesses and infectious disease outbreaks. Few people know that the CDC is also involved in studying diseases related to eating habits, exercise, and smoking. They work with other government agencies and private groups to gather data and produce reports about all factors that affect public health.

Epidemiologists record the incidence of a disease and then plot the information on a map to see whether the disease is occurring in one area or throughout a particular region. It is also important to know the sex, age, and race of the people getting the disease. This helps researchers find any trends that may explain the spread of the disease. For example, it was very important to know that most of the early cases of toxic shock syndrome occurred in menstruating women. This information helped pinpoint one probable cause for toxic shock syndrome. It is also helpful to know other information, such as income, occupation, and personal habits that may affect the individual's health. For example, physicians know that smokers are more susceptible than nonsmokers to respiratory tract infections.

Once epidemiologists detect a disease trend, they must study the rate at which the disease spreads in an area. This information helps them to further detect the way the disease travels from one person to another. It also permits the epidemiologist to predict where the disease may occur next. For example, public health agencies are well aware that bacterial meningitis occurs most commonly among young people in colleges and high schools. This information allows epidemiologists to come up with measures that reduce the spread of meningitis amongst students. Again, it is important to use specific terms to describe the spread of a disease. The **morbidity and mortality rate** represents the percentage of people in a particular population who become ill or die from a particular disease over a specific period of time. The term **incidence** means the number of new cases appearing in a prescribed period. Disease **prevalence** refers to all the cases that appeared over a designated period.

Diseases that regularly occur in a population of organisms are considered endemic. A large number of cases that appear quickly in a particular location define an epidemic. The bacteria causing toxic shock syndrome are responsible for several endemic diseases such as throat and skin infections. At one time, there was a fear that toxic shock syndrome could become epidemic if not controlled. The term **outbreak** refers to epidemics that arise quickly within a specific population of people. Toxic shock syndrome was an outbreak when it was first recognized.

Epidemiologists also study a disease's **mode of transmission. Portal of entry** refers to the surface or body opening where the disease organism enters the body. Related to this term is **portal of exit**, which refers to the surface or body opening where the disease organism leaves the body for possible infection of another person. Toxic shock syndrome has more than one portal of entry and portal of exit. Finally, the term **transmission** describes how the organism arrives at the portal of entry from its previous portal of exit. Understanding the transmission of certain infectious diseases is very difficult if they spread easily by a variety of means. This situation is true for toxic shock syndrome because the disease is transmitted in many ways.

THE EPIDEMIOLOGY OF TOXIC SHOCK SYNDROME

Recall that two different types of bacteria are the main causes of toxic shock syndrome. *Staphylococcus aureus* is responsible for most of the cases, but *Streptococcus pyogenes* also causes the disease. Other bacteria produce conditions similar to toxic shock. These diseases include exanthematous viral syndromes; Gram-negative sepsis; Kawasaki syndrome (a little-known bacterial infection), which is rare in patients older than 4 years; leptospirosis, caused by an organism related to the organism that causes syphilis meningococcemia; and Rocky Mountain spotted fever, which is spread by deer ticks. Sometimes cases of toxic shock syndrome are confused with severe allergic responses to certain drugs. Many of the signs of toxic shock syndrome are allergic reactions to bacterial toxins. Thus, it is understandable that toxic shock syndrome was confused with allergies and other diseases.

Staphylococcal toxic shock syndrome, STSS, was the first type of toxic shock syndrome diagnosed and consequently has the most thorough epidemiological database. Most study of the

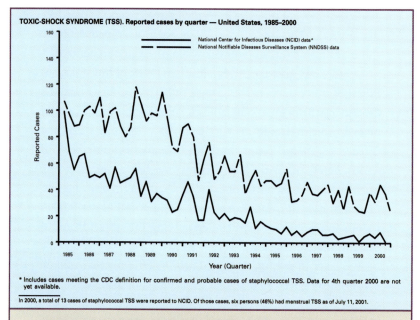

TOXIC-SHOCK SYNDROME (TSS). Reported cases by quarter — United States, 1985–2000

National Center for Infectious Diseases (NCID) data*
National Notifiable Diseases Surveillance System (NNDSS) data

* Includes cases meeting the CDC definition for confirmed and probable cases of staphylococcal TSS. Data for 4th quarter 2000 are not yet available.

In 2000, a total of 13 cases of staphylococcal TSS were reported to NCID. Of those cases, six persons (46%) had menstrual TSS as of July 11, 2001.

Figure 6.1 Scientists learned that certain tampons and the improper use of feminine hygiene products started the toxic shock syndrome outbreak of the 1980s. As can be seen in this graph, incidences of toxic shock syndrome decreased dramatically after 1990, when new regulations and warnings were required for tampon manufacturing and sales.

illness occurred after 1980, when its increased occurrence alerted the medical community to a possible large-scale outbreak (Figure 6.1). The number of cases of toxic shock syndrome recorded between 1970 and 1978 remained consistent at fewer than 200 new cases per year. A lack of knowledge about toxic shock syndrome by the medical community prevented epidemiologists from understanding the true cause of these cases. However, some data showed that one of two strains of *Staphylococcus aureus* caused most of the cases. Over 75 percent of the cases were due to a strain that produced the potent TSST-1 exotoxin described in Chapter 4. The number of cases of toxic shock syndrome grew steadily to approximately 1,200 cases from 1970 to 1980. The CDC recognized this quick rise as an outbreak and carried out an intensive investigation of the disease. It was also at this time that the CDC required all physicians to keep comprehensive records on the disease and report new incidents to the CDC. The death rate, or mortality, from the disease ranged from 3 percent to 6 percent of treated people. The highest mortality occurred early in the outbreak.

The 1980 outbreak of toxic shock syndrome ultimately led to the discovery of the dramatic increase in the disease. The large number of cases provided ample information about the way the bacteria cause toxic shock syndrome and how the organisms spread. Epidemiological studies showed that the incidence of disease went up mostly in women who were menstruating at the time of diagnosis. Over 90 percent of all the TSS cases occurred in females. Menstruating females accounted for 92 percent of the outbreak cases seen in females. The few male patients ranged in age from 1 to 75 years old, whereas the females had a narrower age range clustering around 23 years old. This information led public health officials to suspect a link between **menstruation** and the outbreak. Further investigations revealed that the outbreak resulted from a particular type of tampon used by that age group. Tampons are feminine hygiene products used to prevent the leakage of menstrual fluids during menstruation. Extensive laboratory experiments showed that the tampons were responsible for the increased chance of contracting TSS. Research studies conducted on tampons showed how bacterial growth was fostered by the tampons and encouraged the bacteria to cause toxic shock syndrome. Upon confirming these results, the United States Food and Drug Administration (FDA), stopped the sale certain types of tampon. The FDA also encouraged the labeling of tampons to ensure their use in a manner that reduced the chances of contracting toxic shock syndrome (Figure 6.2).

By 1982, a new investigation into toxic shock syndrome showed a steady decline in the number of cases, to slightly more than 600 newly diagnosed occurrences. Further changes

Ingredients: Rayon and/or cotton fiber, polyethylene/polypropylene overwrap, cotton cord.

Directions for use enclosed.

Tampons come in the following standardized industry-wide absorbencies. Use the chart for comparing absorbencies of all industry products.

The risk of Toxic Shock Syndrome (TSS) increases with higher absorbency. In order to reduce your risk of TSS, you should use the lowest absorbency that meets your needs.

Absorbency Absorbencia	Absorbency Range Niveles de Absorbencia
Regular	6-9 grams/gramos
Super	9-12 grams/gramos
Super Plus	12-15 grams/gramos

Ingredientes: Fibras de rayón y/o algodón, envoltorio de polietileno/polipropileno, cordón de algodón.

Se incluyen las instrucciones de uso.

Los absorbentes internos vienen en los siguientes niveles de absorbencia estandarizados en toda la industria. Vea en la tabla una comparación de absorbencia de todos los productos de la industria.

El riesgo del Síndrome de Choque Tóxico (TSS) aumenta cuando el nivel de absorbencia es mayor. Para reducir el riesgo de TSS, usted debería usar la menor absorbencia que cumpla con sus necesidades.

ATTENTION: TAMPONS ARE ASSOCIATED WITH TOXIC SHOCK SYNDROME (TSS). TSS IS A RARE BUT SERIOUS DISEASE THAT MAY CAUSE DEATH. READ AND SAVE THE ENCLOSED INFORMATION. **ATENCIÓN:** LOS ABSORBENTES INTERNOS ESTÁN ASOCIADOS CON EL SÍNDROME DE CHOQUE TÓXICO (TSS). EL TSS ES UNA ENFERMEDAD POCO COMÚN PERO GRAVE, QUE PUEDE OCASIONAR LA MUERTE. LEA Y GUARDE LA INFORMACIÓN ADJUNTA.

Figure 6.2 The FDA encouraged the labeling of tampons to ensure that they were used in a manner that reduced the chances of contracting toxic shock syndrome. These labels can be found on all tampon boxes. An example of the label is shown in this figure.

in tampon technology resulted in a greater decrease in toxic shock syndrome. These changes caused a dramatic decline between 1982 and 1989. The number of new cases reached the same level of occurrence before 1978. Toxic shock syndrome incidences decreased 10 percent more between 1989 and 1996. The occurrence of the disease then stabilized to fewer than 50 cases a year, the level at which it stands today. Only 71 percent of the toxic shock syndrome cases reported between 1981 and 1986 occurred in menstruating females. The occurrence in menstruating females dropped to 59 percent between 1987 and 1997. Very few cases today are due to tampon use in menstruating females. Public health officials believe that the pattern of decline was due jointly to the improvement of tampons and to public awareness programs. Tampon boxes still carry warning labels, although toxic shock syndrome from tampon use is infrequent today. Public health officials believe that removing the labels could lead to a recurrence of the disease.

It took further study to understand the occurrences of toxic shock syndrome not related to tampon use. Physicians are particularly interested in this information with the development of antibiotic-resistant strains of bacteria. *Staphylococcus aureus* has strains that are resistant to all of the major antibiotics. This can lead to incurable forms of toxic shock syndrome, possibly raising the mortality to 70 percent, as if the disease had run its course untreated. The contagious nature of the bacteria could set in motion an epidemic of *Staphylococcus aureus* diseases.

Scientists did not study streptococcal toxic shock syndrome (StrepTSS) as well during the initial outbreak and subsequent decline of toxic shock syndrome. This was mostly due to its rarity. It took the sharp rise in staphylococcal toxic shock syndrome to alert the medical community to StrepTSS. Most studies indicate that StrepTSS, unlike staphylococcal toxic shock syndrome, is unrelated to tampon use. This led to a new round of epidemiological studies to investigate the causes of StrepTSS. Also unlike staphylococcal toxic shock syndrome, incidences of StrepTSS have been on the rise since 1995. A breakthrough came when medical researchers noted a link between milder *Streptococcus* diseases and an occurrence of StrepTSS. Now physicians pay close attention to patients ailing from *Streptococcus pyogenes* infection, to prevent it from developing into StrepTSS. Several cases of StrepTSS occurring between 1991 and 2000 associated StrepTSS with surgery. This led to a new epidemiology of StrepTSS.

Researchers at the University of Iowa College of Medicine warned physicians in 1991 to watch for StrepTSS in patients after surgery. They noted several incidents of patients developing fevers and rashes resembling StrepTSS. Scientists then confirmed that *Streptococcus pyogenes* could invade surgical wounds that were not clean or were not healing properly. They cautioned that the disease could have a high mortality if not recognized early. Other incidents of StrepTSS occurred after cosmetic or plastic surgery. Another group of studies conducted in 1998 came to the same conclusion about patients having reconstructive surgery involving medical implants. A growth in cosmetic and reconstructive surgery was solely responsible for the increase in what is now termed postoperative StrepTSS. Physicians now have to caution patients about the chance of getting StrepTSS even from simple facelift procedures. Complex surgeries involving breast implants and facial reconstruction are more prone to invasion with *Streptococcus pyogenes*. Unfortunately, the increasing demand for cosmetic surgery produced conditions in which physicians were not performing the surgery under ideal conditions. Consequently, people undergoing cosmetic surgery were more likely to get an infection than patients operated on under better conditions.

OTHER DISEASES CAUSED BY TSS BACTERIA

Staphylococcus aureus and *Streptococcus pyogenes* produce other diseases aside from toxic shock syndrome. Some of these are just as severe as toxic shock syndrome and require the same vigilance to control their spread. Individual differences in humans partly determine how bacteria will behave in the body. People with weakened immune systems will usually suffer more from the effects of bacterial invasion. Chronic disease, excessive alcohol consumption, malnutrition, and stress deteriorate the immune system. The variety of diseases produced by these bacteria also relates to the traits of different strains. *Staphylococcus aureus* has several different strains that lack some of the cell-wall components and secretions produced by the strain causing toxic shock syndrome. These strains produce milder diseases. Yet, some strains are more potent. Almost all *Streptococcus pyogenes* are potentially dangerous because of the many traits used for invading the body. The body more easily combats some strains because they are less able to disarm or destroy the host's immune system. This difference creates conditions in which the damage is restricted to particular regions of the body.

Scalded-skin syndrome (Figure 6.3) is a condition related to staphylococcal toxic shock syndrome. The disease shows the same type of skin damage as toxic shock syndrome. However, it does not spread throughout the body and therefore does not produce a serious fever, kidney damage, or shock. It is most common in babies and children. Few adults show the disease. Most adults who have the disease have a weakened immune system. More mild than scalded-skin syndrome is a condition commonly called "dishpan hands." It is common among people who wash their hands frequently at home or on the job. Continuous handwashing with soap reduces the growth of helpful bacteria, leaving room for *Staphylococcus aureus* to gain control of the skin. Secretions produced by the bacteria irritate the skin, causing reddening and cracking. Certain strains of *Staphylococcus aureus* also cause a skin condition called boils. Boils are pus-filled skin **lesions**. *Staphylococcus aureus* also causes blood vessel inflammation, ear infections, meningitis,

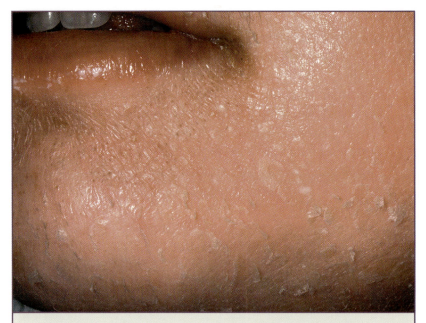

Figure 6.3 Scalded skin syndrome is a severe form of toxic shock syndrome, a result of the *Staphylococcal* form of the disease. The person shown in this picture is suffering from this symptom of the disease, which is most common in babies and children. Note the burned or scalded appearance of the skin.

and pneumonia. It also causes one type of staphylococcal food poisoning. It travels via food handling by people with large populations of *Staphylococcus aureus* on their hands.

Streptococcus pyogenes produces several conditions called **noninvasive streptococcal diseases.** The strains causing these diseases lack some of the secretions needed to penetrate intact tissues. Certain strains of *Streptococcus pyogenes* growing in the throat can cause **pharyngitis.** Pharyngitis is an inflammation of the tonsils and voicebox. Physicians usually call this highly infectious disease "strep throat." *Streptococcus pyogenes* produces approximately 25 percent of the pharyngitis cases.

Scarlet fever is a disease that gained notoriety in nineteenth-century England, when it spread rapidly and killed many people. This *Streptococcus pyogenes* disease usually starts out as pharyngitis, which then progresses to a rash. Severe cases include swelling and damage to the mucous membranes of the respiratory system. Today, it is an uncommon disease that rarely kills people. Mild strains of *Streptococcus pyogenes* produce skin infections such as erysipelas and impetigo. These infectious diseases produce differing degrees of skin rashes. Some of the rashes go deep into the skin and cause swelling of underlying tissues.

Invasive *Staphylococcus aureus* diseases affect areas underlying the mucous membranes and skin. Streptococcal myositis is an inflammation of the muscle tissues near the surface of the body. Scientists believe that the bacteria invade the muscles by entering the body through a throat infection. Sometimes people acquire it through wounds that involve muscle damage. Necrotizing fasciitis is a horrible condition in which *Staphylococcus aureus* freely travels through the tissue underlying the skin. *Staphylococcus aureus* enters this tissue, the fascia, through a wound and rapidly eats away the skin. A sudden increase of cases in the 1990s created a media frenzy. The disease became known as a flesh-eating bacterial infection. *Staphylococcus aureus* can also make its way to the blood, causing a serious condition called bacteremia. The disease kills 40 percent of the people who develop it, and those who do live usually end up with heart damage. *Staphylococcus aureus* is associated with other diseases affecting the joints, kidneys, mouth, and nervous system.

7

Diagnosis and Treatment

We begin to die as soon as we are born, and the end is linked to the beginning.

Manilius, Latin poet, born around 50 B.C.

Death is a common outcome of untreated toxic shock syndrome. Manilius may not see this as an evil outcome of the disease but rather an acceleration of an inevitable fate. Modern physicians cannot accept this interpretation of life and therefore have come up with precise ways of preventing, predicting, diagnosing, and treating toxic shock syndrome and other diseases. Their objective is to save lives and not let the disease run its full course. Death is something to avoid and not welcome with open arms. Before modern medicine, people were at the mercy of diseases, having little recourse other than to suffer and accept the outcomes. Today, most societies can predict how disease occurs and then treat it when it does appear. Ensuring that diseases do not wipe out the human population involves three medical practices called diagnosis, treatment, and prevention.

Diagnosis means identifying a disease and all its causes. This is not always an easy task. Some diseases have the same signs and symptoms leading to an incorrect diagnosis, also known as a misdiagnosis. Toxic shock syndrome resembles other diseases and at first was confused with those conditions. Physicians did not always recognize the disease early in the outbreak of 1981. Alerts by the CDC ensured that physicians would better scrutinize any patient who appeared to have the signs and symptoms of toxic shock syndrome. The fact that toxic shock syndrome can be caused by different bacteria also confounded its diagnosis. So, each diagnosis of toxic shock syndrome required confirmation with an exact identification of the microbe causing that particular case.

Before modern medicine, physicians diagnosed diseases merely by observing the patient's signs and symptoms. The physicians then compared what they observed to a known list of diseases. Today, this type of action is only the initial phase of completing a diagnosis. Physicians now run a series of tests that help identify and isolate the cause in the case of an infectious disease. The tests may include chemical analysis of the blood or tissue samples. It may also involve monitoring kidney function and other body measures, such as blood pressure and heart rate, collectively called vital signs. Usually a sample of the microbe causing a disease is thoroughly examined to ensure that it is not a new strain or type of organism. Diagnosis is only

PREVENTING ILLNESS WITH ILLNESS

The goal of physicians today is to prevent the occurrence and spread of diseases. Most people would agree that it is better not to be sick than to have to get treatment for an illness. It is particularly important that potentially fatal diseases such as toxic shock syndrome are prevented if at all possible. This philosophy of medicine is a complete change from what was practiced up until the 1960s. Many people believed that the best way to prevent serious complications from infectious disease was to be exposed to a mild form of the condition. Many children growing up from the beginning of American history until the 1960s remember having to visit neighbors and family members having childhood diseases. It was known that exposure to people recovering from chicken pox, measles, and mumps produced a mild disease that gave immunity from severe disease. This strategy served the same purpose as variolation. Physicians replaced this way of getting immunity with modern vaccination procedures.

the first step in controlling a disease. It leads to the steps needed for curing a disease.

Treatment means coming up with a strategy for ridding the body of the disease. With infectious diseases such as toxic shock syndrome, treatment means finding a way to kill the offending organism. Medical treatments given before the invention of modern drugs usually involved approaches that rid the body of sin. Most cultures up until the 1900s believed disease was caused by sinful acts. The way to cure disease was to find substances or treatments that cleansed sin from the body. People swallowed or injected substances such as gold or mercury to purify the body or chase away the sin. They also used many herbs to correct imbalances in the body believed to cause the disease. Some of these herbs are used today because they incidentally contain chemicals that relieve the signs and symptoms of disease. Other techniques involved draining the body fluids that may have built up sin or have gotten out of balance with other fluids. It was believed that too much or too little bile caused disease. In addition, it was believed that evil could be removed from the body by draining the blood. Blood was believed to carry sin in the body. Today, we know that disease cures result from removing the specific cause of the disease. This is the strategy used with the treatment of toxic shock syndrome. Physicians prescribe medications to kill the particular organism causing toxic shock syndrome as soon as they identify the type of microbe. They also use other drugs to relieve signs and symptoms that aggravate the disease (Figure 7.1). Treatment alone is not the way to combat a disease. Physicians are always looking for ways to prevent a disease from occurring.

Prevention of a disease relies on epidemiological information. Scientists called epidemiologists study how diseases spread within a population. They evaluate all the conditions that make people susceptible to the disease and come up with strategies to prevent new cases. It is then the job of physicians

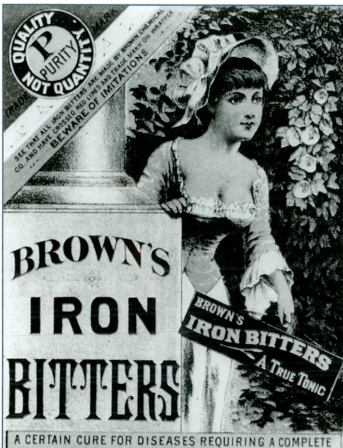

A CERTAIN CURE FOR DISEASES REQUIRING A COMPLETE TONIC, INDIGESTION, DYSPEPSIA, INTERMITTENT FEVERS, WANT OF APPETITE, LOSS OF STRENGTH, LACK OF ENERGY, MALARIA AND MALARIAL FEVERS, &c. REMOVES ALL SYMPTOMS OF DECAY IN LIVER, KIDNEYS AND BOWELS, ASSISTING TO HEALTHY ACTION ALL FUNCTIONS OF THESE GREAT ORGANS OF LIFE. ENRICHES THE BLOOD, STRENGTHENS THE MUSCLES AND GIVES NEW LIFE TO THE NERVES.

BURROW-GILES LITH. CO. N.Y.

Figure 7.1 Throughout modern history, medications were given to get rid of diseases and relieve signs and symptoms that aggravated the condition. This historic advertisement describes a remedy that was used to treat fever, loss of strength and appetite, muscle aches, and indigestion.

and public health officials to apply this information and report new ways that the disease is spreading. Prevention may include reducing certain activities or situations that encourage the spread of a disease. The government developed current food handling and preparation regulations to reduce the proliferation of food-poisoning cases. Improving living conditions has prevented some common diseases of the past. For example, modern sewage disposal reduces the spread of microorganisms that cause digestive system disorders. People maintain their houses today to limit the number of organisms that cause or transmit disease. Better air circulation, regular cleaning of houses, and the storage of food away from pests reduce the spread of disease. Even improvements in personal hygiene can prevent disease. Vaccines are medications developed to prevent the spread of disease. They ensure that the body fends off a harmful microbe before it can cause disease and be passed along to other people.

DIAGNOSIS OF TOXIC SHOCK SYNDROME

Physicians first diagnose toxic shock syndrome by observing the signs and symptoms of the patient suspected of having the disease. However, recall that there are two major causes of toxic shock syndrome. In addition, several diseases such as drug allergies also resemble toxic shock syndrome. Thus, physicians must make a careful assessment of the signs and symptoms before pronouncing a specific diagnosis. The first indication of either form of toxic shock syndrome is a skin rash accompanied by a fever. Fatigue and general body pains help to distinguish toxic shock syndrome from similar ailments. The physician must also investigate any conditions that would point to toxic shock syndrome; they must take into account the patient's age, gender, menstrual cycle, past medical procedures such as surgery, and any other diseases he or she may have at the time. Toxic shock syndrome is very likely to occur in people with AIDS, diabetes, chronic lung diseases, and heart diseases.

Indications of staphylococcal toxic shock syndrome include a fever above 102°F or 39°C and a red, flat rash that covers much of the body. Usually there is also shedding of large sheets of skin on the feet and hands. People with the staphylococcal form of the disease tend to bruise easily and heal slowly. Patients may also display decreased blood pressure and a decrease in urination. Their urine is usually cloudy and filled with cells from the urinary tract. Vomiting and diarrhea commonly accompany the disease, as does a decrease in liver function. Patients usually complain of dizziness, disorientation, fatigue, headaches, and nausea. Special blood tests for staphylococcal antigens and exotoxins can confirm this set of conditions. Physicians will also collect tissue samples to culture for the presence of *Staphylococcus aureus.* Viewing the specimen under a microscope and performing a series of chemical tests will help to identify the bacterium.

Streptococcal toxic shock syndrome is best identified by a red, flat rash covering the body, usually occurring without a fever. Sometimes a low fever occurs, but this is not a common sign of the disease. Another important indicator is a dangerously low blood pressure. The kidneys fail to function and cells cannot get adequate nutrition without proper blood pressure. This very low blood pressure is what usually alerts physicians to the severity of the condition. The low pressure is due to kidney damage, and the patient usually has a reduction of urine production. Shock is very common with streptococcal toxic shock syndrome. Also found with the condition is the characteristic shedding of skin from the feet and hands. Blood tests show clotting problems and decreased liver function. Patients usually complain of breathing difficulties. Tissue samples show exotoxins specific to *Streptococcus.* Cultures which display beta hemolysis and a Lancefield A grouping confirm the presence of *Streptococcus pyogenes.*

Physicians also use epidemiological studies to confirm the diagnosis of toxic shock syndrome. First, they must determine whether the diagnosis of their particular patient is consistent with the population of people who usually get the disease. For example, staphylococcal toxic shock syndrome is mostly associated with females who are menstruating or using certain types of birth control. People who have had recent surgery or severe skin injuries are also subject to staphylococcal toxic shock syndrome. Streptococcal toxic shock syndrome is not limited to one group of people. It is also mostly associated with prior illnesses. People who have had strep throat or streptococcal skin infections are prone to developing streptococcal toxic shock syndrome. Physicians are also alert to streptococcal toxic shock syndrome in patients who have recently undergone cosmetic or reconstructive surgery.

Unfortunately, it may take up to 3 days for confirmation of a particular type of toxic shock syndrome. It takes a couple of days to culture the bacteria and at least a day to conduct all the required medical tests. Quicker and more accurate laboratory methods in development should speed up identification of the bacteria. In addition, companies that produce diagnostic testing equipment are looking into ways that physicians can confirm the presence of the disease using a simple antibody test. These tests are very similar to the pregnancy test kits available at pharmacies and supermarkets. The tests use antibodies to detect the presence of antigens, enzymes, and toxins characteristic of *Staphylococcus aureus* or *Streptococcus pyogenes*. Each test must undergo thorough evaluations for accuracy and consistency before its approval for use in diagnosis. Sometimes this takes several years, depending on the complexity of the test.

TREATMENT OF TOXIC SHOCK SYNDROME

The best treatment of toxic shock syndrome occurs with an accurate diagnosis and confirmation of (Strep TSS and Staph TSS). Physicians have to select a course of treatment specific for the type of toxic shock syndrome. They also must adjust any treatment for the patient's age, degree of health, and medical history. Age is important for determining the amounts of drug to give. Children and the elderly can easily receive overdoses of drugs because their livers and kidneys are less effective at removing excess amounts of drugs from the body. Medical history means any prior diseases or treatments that would affect the treatment of toxic shock syndrome. For example, blood pressure medicine can further damage the kidneys of people with toxic shock syndrome. The physician also must investigate the patient's drug allergies, to ensure that the patient does not become ill from taking a particular medication.

Toxic shock syndrome is treated using a set of actions that kill the bacteria and helps the damaged tissues heal. Treatment also should reduce the chance of other infections taking advantage of the weakened immune system. This is done by giving medications that reduce the spread of other bacteria and fungi. Treatment usually requires hospitalization and continues until the patient is free of the pathogenic bacteria. It is also important that the patient is healthy enough to leave the hospital without getting sick from complications of the disease. Toxic shock syndrome leaves the immune system weakened to the point where a patient can become deathly ill from a cold or sore throat picked up from friends or relatives at home. The patient can also readily pick up pathogens from pets and contaminated food. Regular monitoring of the treatment is needed to ensure that the patient's signs are returning to normal. It is important that the patient does not have any of the symptoms that accompany toxic shock syndrome.

A first step in treating staphylococcal toxic shock syndrome is to decontaminate the areas where the bacteria are growing by removing the bacteria. This removes the enzymes and exotoxins that produce many of the disease's signs and symptoms. The treatment ranges from washing the area with antiseptic soaps to scraping away the infected mucous membranes and skin. Next, the patient is given plenty of fluids to elevate blood pressure and assist kidney function. Many patients need 10 liters, or about 2.5 gallons, of fluid within the first 24 hours of treatment. Then the patient is treated with antibiotics. Antibiotics must destroy all of the offending bacteria while not harming the helpful bacteria. The antibiotic clindamycin is usually the treatment of choice because of the high probability that *Staphylococcus aureus* is resistant to common antibiotics such as penicillin. Minerals and salts given **intravenously** will ensure normal body functions. Properly balanced minerals and salts are needed for heart and nerve function. These minerals and salts get off balance due to abnormal kidney function and the inability to drink. Intensive monitoring then follows the treatment to ensure that disease will not return. Difficult cases receive vaccines that help fight off the effects of the TSST-1 toxin. Sometimes TSST-1 remains in the body and prolongs damage to the body. The vaccine also helps the body to fight off any remaining bacteria. Approximately 3 percent of people treated for staphylococcal toxic shock syndrome die.

The treatment strategy for streptococcal toxic shock syndrome is similar to that for the staphylococcal form. Again, the infected area must be thoroughly cleaned to remove the bacteria and reduce the levels of enzymes and exotoxins. *Streptococcus pyogenes* are very potent. Removing the bacteria and the toxins will reduce further immune system damage. The extreme low blood pressure accompanying streptococcal toxic shock syndrome requires a strict routine of fluid intake. Many patients require at least 20 liters, or about 5 gallons, of fluid a day given intravenously. Special drugs, called *pressors*, are administered along with the fluids, which helps to stabilize blood pressure. Patients need both fluid and pressors to control the extremely low blood pressure that occurs with streptococcal toxic shock syndrome.

Vaccines called *antitoxins* can neutralize toxins if administered early in the treatment of streptococcal toxic shock syndrome. Again, this is due to the potent nature of the toxins. Antibiotic treatment is also an option, although the type of antibiotic used will vary with the strain of *Streptococcus pyogenes* causing the infection. Penicillin can control many of the strains that begin as skin infections. People with penicillin allergies receive alternate treatments of related antibiotics. Clindamycin is the best treatment for strains that start out in the mucous membranes of the throat. Antibiotic treatment continues until the patient's blood indicates no sign of infection. Approximately 30 percent of people treated for streptococcal toxic shock syndrome die.

PREVENTION OF TOXIC SHOCK SYNDROME

Prevention is the preferred way to control both types of toxic shock syndrome. Communications provided by the CDC and local public health agencies alert physicians about any rise in disease prevalence. These alerts make physicians more vigilant about looking for toxic shock syndrome in their areas. It also prepares them to educate patients about ways to prevent the disease. Prevention also involves the identification of high-risk groups. This allows physicians to monitor patients in the high-risk group to catch early indications of toxic shock syndrome. It gives physicians more direction about whom to counsel about the disease

A 2002 information sheet released by the CDC updated its high-risk categories for toxic shock syndrome. They report that menstruating females are three times more likely to get staphylococcal toxic shock syndrome than the rest of the population. They also found that 90 percent of the cases occur in women between 15 and 19 years old. Streptococcal toxic shock syndrome occurs equally in females and males. It appears in all age groups, but it is more common in people between 20 and 59 years old. People who have had recent surgery or skin injuries are more likely to develop streptococcal toxic shock syndrome. It is most likely to appear 2 days after surgery.

WHAT THE PACKAGE SAYS:	ACTUAL ABSORBENCY RANGE:
Junior Absorbency	6 grams and under
Regular Absorbency	6 to 9 grams
Super Absorbency	9 to 12 grams
Super Plus Absorbency	12 to 15 grams

Figure 7.2 Tampon safety studies investigated how the absorbency of tampons was related to toxic shock syndrome. When a tampon that is more absorbent than necessary is used, it increases the chance that harmful bacteria will collect and begin to reproduce. It is best for a woman to use the lowest absorbency possible for her needs. Tampons generally come in four sizes, junior (or light), regular, super, and super plus. The actual absorbency range for each size is shown here.

People with AIDS and weakened immune systems are also very likely to get both forms of toxic shock syndrome.

Staphylococcal toxic shock syndrome became well known because better information about feminine-hygiene devices could have prevented its outbreak. The outbreak of 1980 was solely due to a particular type of tampon that encouraged the growth of *Staphylococcus aureus*. Certain tampons held on to the menstrual fluids in a manner that encouraged the growth of bacteria. Bacteria such as *Staphylococcus* and *Streptococcus* thrive on the body fluids and cells found in the menstrual flow. In addition, people were not fully educated about the risks of using tampons improperly. This led to various studies that investigated tampon safety. The studies confirmed that certain tampon designs raised the risks of staphylococcal toxic shock syndrome. Other studies indicated that educating people about the proper use of tampons reduced the risk of contracting staphylococcal toxic shock syndrome. All of this culminated in government regulations that strictly controlled the development and marketing of feminine-hygiene products (Figure 7.2).

8

Case Study: Toxic Shock and Feminine Hygiene

Man has his will, but woman has her way.

Oliver Wendell Holmes (1809–1894),
from *Autocrat of the Breakfast Table*

Holmes was not completely accurate about women having their way as they please. The onset of puberty brings with it a monthly ritual that they have no control over. This ritual of menstruation causes the female body to shed the lining of its uterus (Figure 8.1). This lining develops into a thick layer of tissue in preparation for pregnancy. If the pregnancy does not occur, the body releases the thickened lining as a flow of blood-like tissue from the female reproductive tract. To control the blood flow, women developed personal hygiene methods to reduce the soiling of clothing from the leakage of menstrual fluids. In 1980, these efforts brought with them an unexpected susceptibility to staphylococcal toxic shock syndrome. Women had little control over the spread of this disease. The design and recommended use of tampons were the main culprits. The following theoretical case study from 1990 dramatizes the seriousness of improperly designed personal-hygiene products and over-the-counter medical devices. It represents a typical case that would have been common between 1978 and 1980 at the height of the toxic shock outbreak related to tampon use.

A 16-year-old female was admitted to hospital with vomiting and a 39.9°C fever. She had been healthy up to 2 days prior to admission.

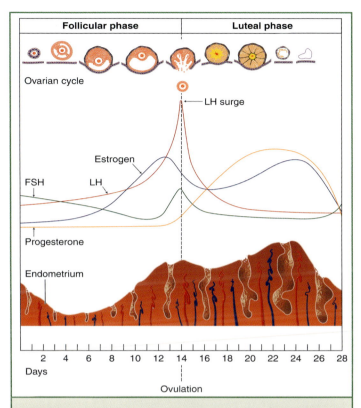

Figure 8.1 During a woman's fertile years, her body prepares for pregnancy once a month by building up the uterine lining. If the woman does not become pregnant, the lining of the uterus is released through the vaginal canal. Women use many methods to absorb and collect the menstrual flow, including tampons. An illustration of the buildup of the uterine lining and the hormones throughout the monthly cycle is shown here.

On the morning of admission, she had diarrhea and a below-normal blood pressure of 76/48 millimeters of mercury [the standard system for measuring blood pressure]. Her heart rate was rapid at 120 beats per minute [normal heart rate for this age group is approximately 80 beats per minute]. She had red rash, which was most prominent on her abdomen. Cultures were obtained from the rash. The patient was immediately given intra-venous fluids and antibiotics. She was monitored in the pediatric intensive care unit. Her laboratory results showed elevated liver enzymes, increased blood urea, and a high white blood cell count at 14,300 cells per mm^3. The patient was reported to have begun her menstrual period 4 days prior to her illness.

It is evident from the signs and symptoms discussed in Chapters 4 and 7 that the patient is suffering from staphylococ-cal toxic shock syndrome. It is possible that her illness was the result of improper tampon use, and could have been avoided if she had been more aware of the necessary precautions. The tampon she used to collect her menstrual flow was designed to reduce the growth of toxic shock syndrome bacteria. Unfortu-nately, even though the tampon was manufactured safe, she used an old tampon and failed to remove it after it became soiled, causing this preventable condition. This case of staphylococcal toxic shock syndrome would have reflected an improperly designed tampon if this had happened in 1980. However, after the 1980s, tampon companies began manufacturing safer tampons, to reduce the chance of a woman contracting TSS from using this common menstrual product. It is possible that the girl in this case study, for some reason, did not follow the advice and warnings required on all feminine-hygiene products since 1982, which led to her condition.

A BRIEF HISTORY OF FEMININE-HYGIENE DEVICES

Menstrual flow has rarely been considered a favorable event throughout human history. Some cultures even required women to hide or isolate themselves from the rest of society during their menstrual flow period. Some cultures collected the flow and discarded it far from away from the community. Some societies have considered menstruating women unclean. Some anthropologists speculate that these taboos about menstrual flow stemmed from a prehistoric fear that the smell of the fluid would attract predators. Bears, large cats, and wolves have a keen sense of smell and are particularly sensitive to the blood and hormones found in menstrual fluids.

Throughout history, women have used various tampon-like devises to catch menstrual fluids. Archeological digs in Egypt showed that the ancient Egyptians created a tampon-like device using rolls of papyrus stems. Papyrus is a large reed that grows wild in wet areas of Egypt. Its soft, thick stems were flattened and rolled into a tough paper. Papyrus is more absorbent than contemporary paper made from softwood trees such as fir and pines. In Africa, many women used rolled grass and leaves of local plants to stop menstrual flow. This practice probably originated in prehistoric times. Japanese physicians favored rolled paper made from trees to collect menstrual fluids. The paper was rough and similar to canvas. Roman women used a more commonly available resource for tampons. Animal materials such as wool and animal hides were favored over paper due to their better durability.

A Colorado physician invented the first modern tampon in the 1930s (Figure 8.2). This simple tampon was made from rolled cotton that females inserted into their vaginal tracts. However, this tampon only lasted on the market for a short period of time due to the scarce availability of cotton and its high prices. To remedy this problem, manufacturers of feminine-hygiene products began replacing cotton with an inexpensive synthetic fiber called rayon. Rayon is a cellulose fiber formed when chlorine bleach mixes with wood pulp, and is just as absorbent as cotton. Rayon and rayon-cotton blends became the most popular tampon filler in the late 1970s. In 1995, some public interest groups raised concerns about the possible presence of toxic compounds in rayon products. One group of compounds, called dioxins, was shown to cause serious tissue irritation and cancer in laboratory animals. Although the dioxin levels in tampons are very low, the average

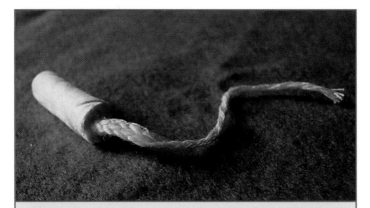

Figure 8.2 Tampons in their modern form were developed in the 1930s. Prior to that, women used various materials including paper, papyrus reeds, and grass to absorb menstrual flow. The first modern tampons were made with rolled cotton that was eventually replaced with the synthetic fiber rayon, made from bleached wood pulp. A modern tampon is shown in this photograph.

woman could use over 10,000 tampons in a lifetime. This could cause a dangerous buildup of dioxins in the body. Additionally, dioxins are easily absorbed by mucous membranes and accumulate for years in the body's fatty tissues.

Rayon is still used in tampons today but is now only one of many synthetic fibers. Most of the new fibers are chemically related to nylon and plastic. These fibers are not as absorbent as the natural cellulose fibers found in cotton and rayon. To remedy this problem, manufacturers placed additives in these products to improve absorbency. Soap-like compounds called *surfactants* were one of the additives placed in tampons. Surfactants produce a barrier that prevents the invasion of bacteria into the menstrual fluids absorbed by the tampon. Eventually, manufacturers added other chemicals, such as fragrances and preservatives, in attempts to improve the product by reducing odors from the menstrual fluids. However, the safety of these synthetic materials and the new additives also raised concern.

The next improvement involved the development of extra-absorbent tampons structured to collect and hold larger amounts of fluid. They leaked less than the standard tampon and required changing less often. Some concerns arose about the use of asbestos in tampons in the late 1980s, as the chemical became known as a hazardous substance. Many people believed that asbestos was used because it is absorbent and does not degrade like cellulose when wet. This concern was just a rumor, however, and never supported by evidence.

Throughout history, tampons have not been the only strategy to deal with menstrual flow. Women in many cultures lined their undergarments with absorbent materials to catch the menstrual fluid. Menstrual pads were first made from absorbent pads of molded cotton sheets. Cotton was replaced by cotton gauze during World War I, as cotton became scarce. Gauze was made from other cellulose products and wool. The Kimberly-Clark company marketed a new product in 1920, naming it Kotex because the material was cotton-textured. Modern menstrual pads contain the same filler materials as tampons, making them more absorbent and less likely for fluid to leak onto clothing.

THE IMPACT OF STSS ON FEMININE HYGIENE

The death of Betty O'Gilvie in Kansas shook up the feminine-hygiene market. She was the most noted of the approximately 3000 women who contracted staphylococcal toxic shock syndrome from tampons use during the 1979–1982 outbreak. She died after using a tampon developed by International Playtex, Incorporated. The courts held the company liable for her death because it had provided only the minimum information needed to convey safety issues regarding tampon use. The company argued that they complied with the FDA's requirements for warning labels on tampons. However, a jury disagreed and awarded O'Gilvie's family $1.35 million. Many people were angry that Playtex did not remove a potentially unsafe product from the market. They felt it was not enough to provide a minimum warning label. Women wanted the confidence that the product would not produce staphylococcal toxic shock syndrome even if used improperly.

This lawsuit followed the Procter & Gamble Rely brand tampons incident of 1980. Research studies conducted by the CDC and several university laboratories linked Rely tampons to the outbreak of staphylococcal toxic shock syndrome. The FDA forced Procter & Gamble to stop manufacturing the

TOXIC SHOCK SYNDROME AND FEMINISM

The first report that linked the increase in toxic shock syndrome to tampons led to renewed activism of the American feminist movement of the 1960s. Feminists argued that tampons were designed more for cosmetic value and not for safety. One argument was that the tampons contained potentially hazardous chemicals solely used to cover up odors. They claimed that odors were not a significant problem. The supposed benefits of eliminating odors were not worth the risks of exposure to the deodorants and fragrances used in the tampons. The feminist perspective was not without merit. Research studies performed by various scientists provided strong evidence that the chemicals used in tampons caused irritation to the vaginal tract. This irritation could make women more susceptible to vaginal tract infections. Their other argument was that tampons encouraged disease by keeping the menstrual fluids in contact with the vaginal lining. This prevented the fluids from draining and encouraged bacterial growth near the sensitive vaginal lining. Again, scientific evidence supported the feminist concern. This research and the toxic shock syndrome outbreak moved the government to set stricter safety regulations for tampon design. It also led to education programs instructing women about the proper use of tampons.

tampons and withdraw any that were still in stores. This action of labeling tampons followed a lawsuit in which Procter & Gamble claimed that the product was safe. It said that the staphylococcal toxic shock syndrome developed from improper tampon use. The courts felt otherwise and forced all feminine-hygiene product manufacturers to prove the safety of their products by conducting extensive clinical tests on animals and humans. The lawsuit also resulted in the 1982 FDA regulation requiring warning labels on tampon boxes. However, the warning labels were not meant to cover up the continued manufacturing of dangerous products, as the O'Gilvie versus International Playtex, Incorporated lawsuit determined. The warnings are meant to warn women about the potential problems that could occur with improper tampon use.

The recall of potentially dangerous tampons significantly reduced the incidence of new staphylococcal toxic shock syndrome cases. By 1986, the number of cases returned to just above the normal incidence of staphylococcal toxic shock syndrome. The greatest decrease occurred when companies pulled old tampons from the shelves and replaced them with ones that did not foster the growth of *Staphylococcus aureus*. Many types of bacteria thrive in the nutrient-rich menstrual fluids. Tampons that stored large amounts of the fluid became incubators for *Staphylococcus aureus*. It took much experimentation to develop products that were highly absorbent but did not encourage the growth of bacteria. In addition, researchers discovered that certain filler materials, such as polyacrylate, stimulated the growth of bacteria. This was compounded by the fact that women were more likely to keep such tampons inserted longer than less absorbent ones. Therefore, the tampon provided a way for large amounts of *Staphylococcus aureus* to come in contact with the sensitive mucous membranes of the vagina. In addition, the highly absorbent tampons dried the vaginal lining, increasing the possibility of tiny tears in the lining and making it easier for *Staphylococcus aureus* to invade the body.

Glossary

Acquired—A disease term meaning that a condition is picked up from a chemical, object, or organism.

Adhesin—Proteins that permit cells to stick to other cells.

Aerobic—Requiring oxygen to carry out life processes.

Allergy—A condition in which the body produces an abnormally strong response to combating disease.

Anaerobic—Does not require oxygen to carry out life processes.

Antibiotic—A drug used to kill or slow down the growth of bacteria.

Antibiotic resistant—Having characteristics that render bacteria impervious to toxic effects of antibiotics.

Antibody—Chemicals produced by the immune system that are used to fight disease.

Antigen—A chemical that stimulates the immune system.

Autoimmune disease—A condition in which the body accidentally uses the immune system to attack itself.

Bacteria—A large group of simple microscopic organisms composed of one cell. Singular is **bacterium**.

Black plague—Also known as bubonic plague, an infectious disease caused by the bacterium *Yersinia pestis* and spread by the bite of rat fleas and by direct contact with infected individuals.

Catheter—A tube inserted through the skin or into a body opening.

Cell—The smallest fundamental unit of living structure composing all organisms.

Cellular—Pertaining to cells or the activities and functions of cells.

Cell wall—A covering surrounding a cell using found in bacteria, fungi, and plants.

Chemoorganotroph—Bacteria that obtain energy by eating decaying organisms.

Cluster—A group of bacteria with similar characteristics.

Coagulase—A bacterial enzyme that causes blood cells to clot.

Cocci—Cells shaped like spheres.

Complements—Proteins produced by the immune system that aid in the removal of disease organisms.

Contagious—A disease condition that can readily spread from one organism to another.

Diagnosis—A medical term describing the identification and naming of a disease.

Digestive tract—A tube running from the mouth to the rectum used for digesting and taking up nutrients from food.

Disease—Any condition that causes illness or produces abnormal effects in the body.

Domesticate—To raise animals or plants that serve the purposes of people.

Emergent disease—A rare condition or disease that becomes very common with the potential of spreading worldwide.

Encephalitis—A disease marked by inflammation of the brain.

Enterotoxins—A group of poisons, produced by intoxicant bacteria, that cause disease signs and symptoms. Many of these poisons reside in the digestive tract of the host.

Enzymes—Proteins that carry out certain functions for an organism. Enzymes perform chemical reactions needed for digestion and metabolism.

Epidemiology—The study of the causes and spread of disease.

Exotoxins—Bacterial secretions that cause disease in host organisms of pathogenic bacteria.

Ferment—To breakdown chemicals using anaerobic processes.

Glossary

Fermentation—The breakdown of chemicals by anaerobic microorganisms.

Fungi—A plant-like microscopic organism that feeds on decaying matter and living organisms.

Hemolysins—Microbial enzymes that cause hemolysis, or the breakdown, of red blood cells.

Hemolysis—The breakdown of red blood cells.

Host—An organism whose body serves as a place for an invading creature to live to obtain protection or food.

Immune system—A complex system of body parts and cells that help recognize and fight off disease. Certain cells of the immune system produce antibodies.

Immunosuppression—A condition in which the immune system fails to function properly.

Infectants—Organisms whose sole presence produces disease.

Infection—Invasion of the body by a disease organism.

Infectious—The ability of a disease to spread throughout the body and from one organism to another.

Inflammation—A reaction to injury involving pain, reddening, and swelling.

Incidence—The number of new cases appearing in a prescribed period.

Innate immunity—See Nonspecific immunity.

Intoxicants—Organisms that produce secretions specifically designed to cause disease for their own survival.

Intravenous—Fluids or medications placed directly into the veins of a person.

Invasive treatment—A medical treatment that involves opening the skin or inserting something into a body opening.

Leprosy—A chronic, communicable bacterial disease of the nervous system caused by *Mycobacterium leprae*. Also called Hansen's disease.

Leptospirosis—An infectious urinary tract condition caused by the spirochete bacterium *Leptospira*.

Lesion—An open sore on the skin or internal body parts.

Lyme disease—An inflammatory disease caused by the bacterium *Borrelia burgdorferi* spread by the bite of certain ticks.

Lymphatic tissue—Tissues such as lymph nodes, tonsils, and lymphatic vessels that make up a large component of the immune system.

Macrophages—Large white blood cells that swallow and destroy foreign matter, including microorganisms.

Menstruation—The monthly release of the uterine lining from the female reproductive tract. The uterine lining is produced to prepare the uterus for pregnancy and is shed if pregnancy does not occur.

Microbe—Same as microorganism. A microscopic organism is usually composed of one cell. Bacteria, fungi, protozoa, and viruses are microorganisms.

Microbiologist—A scientist who studies microorganisms such as algae, bacteria, molds, and protozoa.

Microorganism—A small organism that requires the use of a microscope to be seen. Algae, bacteria, molds, and protozoa are microorganisms.

Mode of transmission—The way a disease spreads from one host to another.

Morbidity rate—The number of people made ill by a disease in a certain period of time.

Mortality rate—The number of people killed by a disease in a certain period of time.

Mucous membrane—A moist, mucus-covered tissue lining the digestive, respiratory, reproductive, and urinary systems.

Mucus—A thick, sticky fluid produced by mucous membranes.

Noninvasive streptococcal diseases—A variety of diseases of of the skin and mucous membranes caused by *Streptococcus* bacteria that cannot invade the body.

Glossary

Nonspecific immunity—Protection against general pathogens. Another name for innate immunity.

Opportunistic disease—A disease caused by an organism that normally does not cause harm.

Organism—A living individual such as an animal, mold, or a plant.

Outbreak—A nonmedical term meaning the sudden occurrence of many cases of a disease.

Pathogen—An organism that causes disease in another organism.

Pharyngitis—Inflammation of the membranes of the nose and upper throat.

Pink eye—An eye infection in cattle and humans caused by the *Hemophilus* bacterium.

Polio—A shortened term for the viral disease poliomyelitis. It causes damage to the nervous system.

Portal of entry—The surface or body opening where the disease organism enters the body.

Portal of exit—The surface or body opening where the disease organism leaves the body.

Prevalence—All the cases of a disease that appear over a designated period.

Protozoan—A microscopic, single-celled organism. Amoebae and the organism causing malaria are protozoans.

Pus—A fluid resulting from an infection. It contains white blood cells, immune system fluids, and infectious microorganisms.

Pyogenic—The ability to produce pus.

Pyrogen—A fever-inducing chemical produced by the body or by microorganisms.

Pyrogenic—The ability to produce fever.

Reproductive tract—All the external and internal parts of females and males used in reproduction. It shares parts with the urinary system.

Respiratory system—A body system for exchanging blood gases with the environment. The lungs, nose, respiratory tree, and throat are parts of the respiratory system.

Rocky Mountain spotted fever—An infectious disease caused by a bacterium-like organism called *Rickettsia*. It spreads throughout the body, and transmission occurs through tick bites.

Scalded-skin syndrome—A bacterial disease condition that shows the same type of skin damage as toxic shock syndrome.

Secretions—A substance produced by cells or microorganisms made to flow out of the cell or organism.

Sepsis—The presence of microorganisms throughout the body, spread by the bloodstream.

Septic diseases—A broad group of diseases caused by pathological microorganisms invading the body, usually through the bloodstream.

Septicemia—The presence of microorganisms in the bloodstream.

Serotyping—A test that uses antibodies to determine different strains of bacteria.

Shock—A condition in which the body collapses and has difficulty functioning. Shock may be due to low blood pressure from extreme blood loss or disease.

Sign—A disease term. A condition that the physician can measure or see during diagnosis. Redness, sores, and swelling are examples of disease signs.

Smallpox—A highly infectious viral disease that scars the skin and internal organs.

Spirochete—A group of spiral-shaped bacteria that cause disease in a variety of organisms. Spirochetes cause leptospirosis, Lyme disease, and syphilis.

Staphylococcus aureus—A pathogenic skin and nasal bacterium that can cause staphylococcal toxic shock syndrome.

Staphylococcal toxic shock syndrome—A destructive disease of the body caused by a bacterium called *Staphylococcus aureus*.

Glossary

Strain—A variation of one type of organism.

Streptococcus pyogenes—A pathogenic skin bacterium that can cause streptococcal toxic shock syndrome.

Streptococcal toxic shock syndrome—A destructive disease of the body caused by a bacterium called *Streptococcus pyogenes.*

Superantigens—Chemicals produced by intoxicant bacteria that cause disease signs and symptoms. They stimulate a strong immune response in the hosts of pathogens.

Symptom—A disease term. A subjective condition due to the patient's feelings. Dizziness, headache, nausea, and pain are examples of disease symptoms.

Syndrome—A complex series of conditions that produce a disease. Syndromes involve disease in many body organs.

Tampon—A feminine-hygiene device inserted into the vaginal tract to absorb menstrual flow.

Therapeutic—Regarding a treatment for curing or lessening a disease.

Tissue—A group of cells in the body that carry out a specific body function. Tissues make up body organs, such as nerve tissue making up the brain.

Trait—Characteristics of an organism, such as its color, shape, size, and means of obtaining food energy.

Transmission—The spread of a disease.

Trauma—Damage to the body, such as a bruise or a wound.

TSST-1—Toxic shock syndrome toxin 1. An exotoxin produced by *Staphylococcus aureus.*

Urbanization—The construction of cities having large populations living in a small area.

Urinary tract—Organs associated with the production and removal of urine wastes.

Variolation—The process of taking pus or scab material from one infected individual and introducing it into a scratch or cut in the skin of another individual to induce immunity. First used to protect against smallpox.

Virulence factors—Characterists of a organism that help it produce disease in a host.

Virus—A very small infectious agent that can only live within the cells of other organisms.

Zoonoses—Diseases spread from animals to humans.

Bibliography

Bauman R. *Microbiology*. San Francisco: Pearson Education. 2002.

Barry, W., L. Hudgins, S.T. Donta and E.L. Pesanti. "Intravenous immuno-globin therapy for toxic shock syndrome." *Journal of the American Medical Association*. 267(1992):3315-3316.

Beers, M.H. and R. Berkow (eds). "Bacterial disease: toxic shock syndrome." *The Merck Manual of Diagnosis and Therapy* accessed online at http://www.merck.com/pubs/mmanual/section13/chapter157/157a.htm.

Berkow, R., M.H. Beers, A.J. Fletcher and R.M. Bogin (eds). "Coccal infections: toxic shock syndrome." *The Merck Manual of Medical Information* accessed online at http://www.merck.com/pubs/mmanual_home/sec17/178.htm.

Broome, C.V. "Epidemiology of toxic shock syndrome in the United States." *Review of Infectious Diseases*. 11(1989):S14-S21.

Centers for Disease Control and Prevention. "Case definition for public health surveillance in the United States." *Morbidity and Mortality Weekly Report*. 39(1990):38-39.

Chesney, P.J., J.P. Davis, W.K. Purdy, P.J. Wand and R.W. Chesney. "Clinical manifestations of toxic shock syndrome." *Journal of American Medical Association*. 246(1981):741-748.

Colbry, S.L. "A review of toxic shock syndrome: the need for education still exists." *Nurse Practitioner*. 17(1992):40-46.

Cunningham, M.W. "Pathogenesis of group A streptococcal infections." *Clinical Microbiology Reviews*. 13(2000):470-511.

Dhawan, V.K. "Toxic shock syndrome." *EMedicine Journal*. 3(2002):1-23.

Dierauf, L.A. and F.M. Guiland. *CRC Handbook of Marine Mammal Medicine*. Pittsburgh, Pa.: CRC Press. 2001.

Friedman, N. *Everything you must know about tampons*. New York: Berkley Publishing, 1981.

Hajjeh, R.A., A. Reingold, W. Alexis, K. Shutt, A. Schuchat and B.A. Perkins. "Toxic shock syndrome in the United States: surveillance update, 1979-1996." *Emerging Infectious Diseases Report*. 6(2000). Accessed at http://www.cdc.go/ncidod.eid/vol5no6/hajjeh.htm.

Houppert, K. "Embarrassed to death: the hidden dangers of the tampon industry." *Village Voice*. February (1995):31-40.

Hribalova, V. "Streptococcus pyogenes and the toxic shock syndrome." *Annals of Internal Medcine*. 108(1988):772.

Lauter, C.B. "Recent advances in toxic shock syndrome." *Contemporary Internal Medicine.* 6(1994):11-22.

List of Bacterial Names with Nomenclature for *Staphylococcus*: http://www.bacterio.cict.fr/s/staphylococcus.html.

List of Bacterial Names with Nomenclature for *Streptococcus*: http://www.bacterio.cict.fr/s/streptococcus.html.

Manders, S.M. "Toxin-mediated streptococcal and staphylococcal disease." *Journal of the American Academy of Dermatology.* 39(1998):383-397.

Michigan Department of Community Health. Communicable disease case definitions and history forms accessed at http://www.michigan.gov/mdch/0,01607,7-132-2945-13855—,00.html.

Nester, E.W., D.G. Anderson, C.E. Roberts, N.N. Pearsall, and M.T Nester. *Microbiology: A Human Perspective.* New York: McGraw-Hill. 2001.

Schlievert, P.M. "Comparison of cotton and cotton/rayon tampons for effect on production of toxic shock syndrome toxin." *Journal of Infectious Diseases.* 172(1992):1112-1114.

Schuchat, A. "Group B streptococcus." *Lancet.* 353 (1999):51-56.

Schuchat, A. and C.V. Broome. "Toxic shock syndrome and tampons." *Epidemiology Review.* 13(1991):99-112.

Seeley, R.R., T.D. Stephans and P. Tate. *Essentials of Anatomy and Physiology.* New York: WCB McGraw-Hill. 1999.

Shands, K.N., G.P. Schmid and B.B. Dan. "Toxic shock syndrome in menstruating women." *New England Journal of Medicine.* 303(1980):1436-1442.

Tofte, R.W. and D.N. Williams. "Clinical and laboratory manifestations of toxic shock syndrome." *Annuals of Internal Medicine.* 96(1982):843-847.

"Toxic Shock Syndromes." United States National Library of Medicine. National Institutes of Health. Medicineplus Medical Encyclopedia accessed at http://www.nlm.nih.gov/medicineplus/enxy/article/000653.htm.

Further Reading

Bauman, R. *Microbiology.* San Francisco; Pearson Education. 2002.

D'Arcy, Jorgensen A. *Toxic Shock Syndrome: The Controversy.* Belmont, Calif.: PPI Publishers. 1985.

Friedman, N. *Everything you must know about tampons.* New York: Berkley Publishing, 1981.

Nester, E.W., D.G. Anderson, C.E. Roberts, N.N. Pearsall and M.T. Nester. *Microbiology: A Human Perspective.* New York: McGraw-Hill. 2001.

Parker, J.N. *The Official Patient's Sourcebook on Toxic Shock Syndrome.* San Diego, Calif.: Icon Group International. 2002.

Shier, D., J. Butler and R. Lewis. *Essentials of Human Anatomy and Physiology.* New York: McGraw-Hill. 2000.

Centers for Disease Control and Prevention
http://www.cdc.gov

eMedicine–Instant Access to the Minds of Medicine website
http://www.emedicine.com

Health A to Z
http://www.healthatoz.com

HealthLink
http://healthlink.mcw.edu

Health World Online
http://www.healthy.net

Toxic Shock Syndrome Information Service
http://www.tssis.com

Toxicshock.net
http://www.toxicshock.net

World Health Organization
http://www.who.int

Index

Index

Index

Picture Credits

9: © Archivo Iconografico, S.A./CORBIS

13: Data from *Morbidity and Mortality Weekly Report* (MMWR), Vol.49, No. 53, June 14, 2002

15: © MAPS.com/CORBIS

21: © Dr. Gary Gaugler/Visuals Unlimited

22: © Dr. David M. Phillips/Visuals Unlimited

26: Lambda Science Artwork

30: © Mediscan/Visuals Unlimited

36: Courtesy CDC, Public Health Image Library (PHIL)

38: © Bettmann/CORBIS

39: Lambda Science Artwork

44: Lambda Science Artwork

50: © Dr. Gary Gaugler/Visuals Unlimited

52: © "Gladden Willis, MD"/ Visuals Unlimited

57: © David Phillips/Visuals Unlimited

63: © Dr. Richard Kessel & Dr. Gene Shih /Visuals Unlimited

69: Lambda Science Artwork

70: Courtesy CDC, PHIL

76: Courtesy CDC, MMWR, Vol. 49, No. 53, June 14, 2002

78: © Noelle Nardone

82: © Mediscan/Visuals Unlimited

87: National Library of Medicine

94: Information from the FDA

97: Lambda Science Artwork

100: © Noelle Nardone

Cover: © Dr. Gary Gaugler/Visuals Unlimited

About the Author

Brian Shmaefsky is a professor of biology and environmental sciences at Kingwood College near Houston, Texas. He did his undergraduate studies in biology at Brooklyn College in New York and completed masters and doctoral studies at Southern Illinois University at Edwardsville. His research emphasis is in environmental physiology. Dr. Shmaefsky has many publications on science education, some appearing in *American Biology Teacher* and the *Journal of College Science Teaching*. He regularly consults on general biology and microbiology textbook projects. Dr. Shmaefsky actively serves on environmental awareness and policy committees in Texas. He has two children Kathleen, 11, and Timothy, 13, and lives in Kingwood, Texas with his dog Dusty.

About the Editor

The late I. Edward Alcamo was a Distinguished Teaching Professor of Microbiology at the State University of New York at Farmingdale. Alcamo studied biology at Iona College in New York and earned his M.S. and Ph.D. degrees in microbiology at St. John's University, also in New York. He had taught at Farmingdale for over 30 years. In 2000, Alcamo won the Carski Award for Distinguished Teaching in Microbiology, the highest honor for microbiology teachers in the United States. He was a member of the American Society for Microbiology, the National Association of Biology Teachers, and the American Medical Writers Association. Alcamo authored numerous books on the subjects of microbiology, AIDS, and DNA technology as well as the award-winning textbook *Fundamentals of Microbiology*, now in its sixth edition.